THE LITTLE BOOK OF

BABY
MASSAGE

THE LITTLE BOOK OF

BABY MASSAGE

Use the power of touch
to calm your baby

JO KELLETT

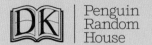

Editor Megan Lea
Senior Designer Collette Sadler
Project Art Editor Louise Brigenshaw
Designers Amy Child, Mandy Earey
Producer, Pre-production David Almond
Senior Producer Luca Bazzoli
Senior Jacket Designer Nicky Powling
Jacket Coordinator Lucy Philpott
Creative Technical Support Sonia Charbonnier
Managing Editor Dawn Henderson
Managing Art Editor Marianne Markham
Art Director Maxine Pedliham
Publishing Director Mary-Clare Jerram

Illustrated by Peter Bull
Photography by Ruth Jenkinson

This book is dedicated to my babies, Alice and Charlie

First published in Great Britain in 2020 by
Dorling Kindersley Limited
80 Strand, London WC2R 0RL

DISCLAIMER see page 144

A CIP catalogue record for this book is available from the British Library.

ISBN: 978-0-2414-1237-4

Printed and bound in China

A WORLD OF IDEAS:
SEE ALL THERE IS TO KNOW

www.dk.com

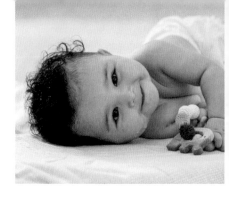

CONTENTS

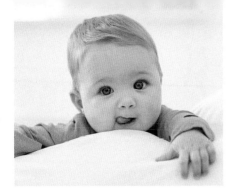
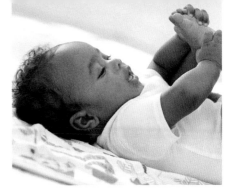

FOREWORD

I came to baby massage whilst pregnant with my first child. I was already an established aromatherapist, working closely with pregnant women, and it seemed a natural progression to train as an infant massage practitioner. Research shows us that holding and caressing a baby is a wonderful way to encourage them to grow up healthy and happy. In many cultures baby massage is routinely carried out as an everyday aspect of childcare; I'm very happy to see it being adopted more and more around the world, as we collectively rediscover the importance of early nurturing for our babies.

I have been teaching baby massage for over 20 years now. It's been a privilege and a wonderful experience to see so many babies and their carers enjoy the process. I have had parents return with their second, and in some cases third, babies. I have also massaged my own two children since birth – they continue to request regular massages, even though they are now in their late teens and early twenties!

We are a tactile species; as babies we need to be carried and held by our parents or carers, for communication, bonding, and health. Massage is an amazing way to teach our children the power of positive touch. This book will allow you to explore that power through a set of routines designed for a range of situations, so you can choose what you think is best for your baby. Massage can be magical for both of you – a time to bond, soothe, relax, and nurture. I sincerely hope you enjoy the process!

Jo Kellett

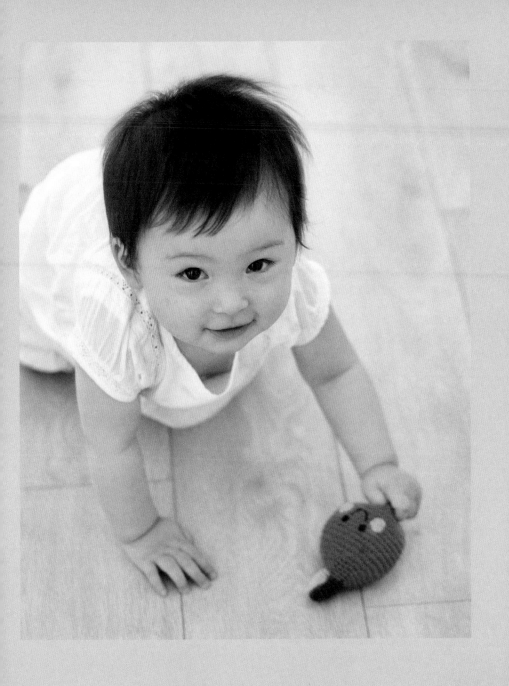

GETTING
STARTED

THE BENEFITS OF BABY MASSAGE

Humans are a tactile species; we need to touch each other to connect, communicate, and thrive. Here are some of the benefits of incorporating baby massage into your routine.

BONDING

Massage is an ideal way to establish a strong bond between you and your baby, through positive touch, eye contact, and vocal assurance. Touch is of prime importance in the bonding process. In addition, during massage your baby is usually face to face with you, making it the perfect opportunity to establish eye contact – babies are drawn to faces, and will search out your eyes.

RELAXATION AND SLEEP

Babies who are massaged regularly appear more relaxed, can be soothed more quickly by being touched, and respond well to touch in stressful situations. Massaging your baby will also be a relaxing experience for you! A massage before bed will make your baby feel loved and encourage them to fall asleep. Regular baby massage may also lead to higher levels of melatonin, the hormone that helps us sleep. See page 76 for a bedtime massage routine.

A BOOST TO THE IMMUNE SYSTEM

Research has shown that massage increases our production of T cells, the white blood cells that help us fight infection. Regular massage may go some way towards keeping our immune system working at its best; it has also been shown to help the initial development of the immune system in babies.

IMPROVED CIRCULATION AND HEALTHY SKIN

Regular massage will help keep your baby's blood circulation in good working order, which in turn helps improve skin tone and texture (see page 104). Massage is also the perfect way to apply moisturisers or lotions to your baby's skin.

BODY AWARENESS

A baby's nervous system is not fully developed at birth. By stimulating the nerve endings in your baby's skin you are helping to teach them body awareness – including giving them a sense of how their limbs are connected to their body.

IMPROVED DIGESTION

Massaging your baby's tummy in a clockwise direction helps with the natural flow of digestion, easing symptoms of colic and constipation (see page 88).

CONFIDENCE

Baby massage helps you feel more sure of your ability to physically handle your baby. By learning a massage routine, and repeating it regularly, you will develop a confident touch outside of massage, which will feel both positive and nurturing to your baby.

NEED TO KNOW

Most parents will use touch to soothe and communicate with their baby without even thinking about it – a massage routine is simply a more structured set of strokes and caresses for you to explore.

Regular massage – daily if possible – is wonderfully beneficial for babies during their early months. A full-body routine should take around 20 minutes to complete, but be guided by your baby; they might only tolerate a few minutes at first, or you may wish to spend longer. Take it slowly, and learn together. To get the full beneficial effects of a massage your baby should be undressed, ideally without a nappy on. However, it's also fine to massage over clothes and without oil if you're in a situation where you can't or don't wish to undress your baby. Baby massage is very different from adult massage. Babies do not hold tension in their muscles as we do. Rather, baby massage is a tool for gentle communication and physical stimulation. When you are learning the routine, start with softer strokes, though don't be too light – even babies find a tickly touch unsettling. Use smooth strokes to convey a sense of confidence that will relax your baby and make them feel secure.

WHEN TO START

If you wish, you can start using the sequences in this book when your baby is as little as a few days old. And if you both enjoy massage, there's no reason not to continue through your baby's first few years and early childhood. As your baby grows and becomes more active, you can reduce how often you massage them to just once or twice a week. If your baby is used to regular massage, maintaining the routine as they start to explore the world around them with more movement allows them to keep reaping the benefits.

A BABY'S BEHAVIOURAL STATES

Newborn babies have six behavioural states, ranging from deep sleep to crying. As you get to know your baby you will recognize these stages and understand their needs. The best time for massage is during the quiet alert phase. This is when your baby is still and fully awake. They are most aware of their surroundings in this state, will focus on objects close by, and will be listening to sounds around them.

KNOWING WHEN NOT TO MASSAGE

Whilst most babies will enjoy and respond positively to massage most of the time, it is important to keep in mind that massage is not always appropriate. If you have any concerns over health issues and whether or not it is right to proceed with massage, speak to your health visitor or GP.

Do not massage your baby if they have a fever or temperature. Nobody likes to be touched when they are feeling poorly. The body feels achy and touch can make your baby feel worse.

If your baby has just been vaccinated, avoid touching the area of the injection site, which can often be slightly raised and inflamed. If your baby has a temperature after vaccination, avoid massage until their temperature goes back to normal. Then

proceed as usual, avoiding the injection site if still raised until it subsides.

If during a massage your baby starts showing signs that they are not happy, such as wriggling excessively or even crying or fussing, then stop. The best way to deal with this is to take a moment to reconnect. Take a deep breath and place your hands over your baby's tummy or chest, making eye contact and talking to them in a soothing voice. It's okay to ask your baby what is wrong, and to encourage them to let you know in their own way. Part of the bonding process is learning to communicate with each other so as to understand your baby's needs.

It's also very important that you are relaxed and have time to perform the massage routine – there's no point in trying to squeeze it into a busy day. Babies very often pick up on your signals and feelings, so if you are feeling stressed it's best to leave massage for another time.

THINGS YOU'LL NEED

You don't need special equipment for baby massage – in fact,
you will almost certainly have most of what you need
at your fingertips already.

VEGETABLE OIL

During massage your hands should glide over your baby's skin with no dragging or resistance, so use an oil or moisturizer. You can either use whatever moisturizer you are currently using on your baby or source a suitable oil. Vegetable oils are best as they are full of vitamins and nourish the skin. Because babies tend to put their fingers in their mouths quite frequently, the oil you use should be as natural as possible, with little or no added fragrance or colouring. This is best purchased from a health food store rather than your local supermarket; choose an oil that is labelled as cold pressed and unfragranced. A cold-pressed sunflower oil is ideal. If you have allergy concerns, avoid oils that come from a nut source, and consult your GP if you are unsure.

Avoid mineral-based oils, which are derived from petroleum: they have no therapeutic properties for your baby's skin, and come from an unsustainable source. What's more, they can sit on the skin, forming a greasy layer instead of being absorbed.

Apply oil as needed during a massage; if you feel any resistance when you stroke across your baby's skin, pour a little more oil into your hands. Always start with just a small amount of oil and add more if you need to – this is easier than using too much and having to wipe it off.

CHANGING MAT, TOWELS, AND WIPES

A changing mat with a towel laid over it placed on the floor is the ideal surface for baby massage. Have spare towels to hand, in case you need to replace the one you are using. An extra towel is also useful for placing over areas of your baby that you have finished massaging to keep your baby warm. Keep wipes, cotton wool, or tissues nearby.

TOYS OR DISTRACTIONS

It's fine for your baby to hold a toy or a soother while you massage them if it makes them feel more comfortable.

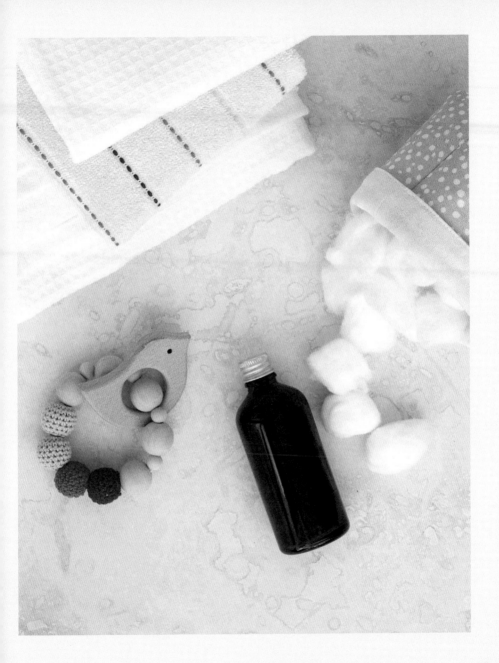

SETTING UP

Once you have everything you need, it's time to get comfy. Here is how to set up the space and position yourself and your baby in preparation for baby massage.

PREPARING FOR MASSAGE

The space where you will give your baby their massage should be warm. For a full-body massage (see page 18) you will need to undress your baby, and applying oil will cool down their skin considerably. Make the room as warm as you can by heating it ahead of massage time, if necessary. Remove all jewellery before you begin, placing it out of your baby's reach, and make sure your fingernails are short and neat.

Sit on the floor and make yourself comfortable with a cushion under your bottom to provide support. Put a towel on top of a changing mat on the floor, then lay your baby in front of you on their back.

If you can't sit comfortably on the floor, place your baby on the surface that you change their nappy on. Don't leave your baby unattended on a raised surface. For sections of the massage where you are massaging your baby's back, you can either lay your baby in front of you with their feet nearest you, or sit with your legs together out in front of you and place your baby on your outstretched legs.

NEWBORN BABIES

If you are massaging a newborn, you may want to sit on the floor with your legs out in front of you, knees apart and feet together (known as "tailor pose" in yoga). Sit with your back supported, against a wall for instance, then bend your knees and bring the soles of your feet together. Place a pillow or blanket between your legs and lay your baby down on it, on their back. When doing strokes that require your baby to lie on their front, bear in mind that very young babies may only be happy in that position for a minute or two.

Babies have a reflex called the tonic neck reflex, sometimes also called the fencing reflex. When they lie on their back their head will turn to one side, the arm on that side may extend, and the arm on the other side tends to bend up towards the head, as if fencing. This reflex shouldn't impede massage and usually disappears when your baby is between 4–7 months old.

MUSIC AND SOUNDS

You may wish to have music playing during a massage: if so, choose something that you and your baby find relaxing. It's also a good idea to talk or even sing to your baby while you massage them. When talking to a baby, most people use a type of speech known as infant-directed speech, or "motherese". This involves using a sing-song tone and shorter words, which are often repeated. Babies respond well to this type of speech, and research suggests that infants are better able to grasp the message when spoken to like this – so if you are already doing it, keep it up during massage!

TOP-TO-TOE MASSAGE

TOP-TO-TOE MASSAGE

A full-body massage can be a rewarding, relaxing way to spend time with your baby. This chapter takes you through a full massage sequence, focusing in turn on each area of your baby's body.

INTRODUCING BABY MASSAGE

As natural as massage feels, it will be a new experience for your baby, so take your time getting into it. Your baby will already be used to you touching their legs through contact during nappy changing, making them a great place to start your exploration of baby massage and gently introduce your baby to the concept. Then, as you both get used to it, have a go at some of the other sequences within the full-body routine. You can either do the whole sequence, or dip in and out – whatever you and your baby prefer!

Start with about five minutes of massage time; as you progress through the routine you will need to put aside more time. Aim for a full-body massage to last approximately 15–20 minutes – though if your baby is happy, you can massage them for longer. It is also perfectly fine to do a shorter routine, or just some of the full-body routine.

YOUR ROUTINE

Finding the right time to massage your baby is crucial. Mid-morning, when your baby is quiet but alert, is often a good time. You may be tempted to jump straight into a massage at bedtime, but it is more important to start by choosing a time when you don't feel under pressure or rushed, and when neither you nor your baby are too tired! As your confidence grows you can use the routine when you want – turn to page 56 for massage sequences tailored to particular times in your day.

BEFORE YOU BEGIN

Make sure the room is warm, and have everything you need to hand so that you don't need to stop during the massage.

Before you start, take a few deep, calming breaths, roll your shoulders to relax them, and rub your hands together to warm them up. It's better to keep contact once you've started – this will encourage a more relaxed experience for you both. Always finish with a cuddle. Most of all, enjoy it!

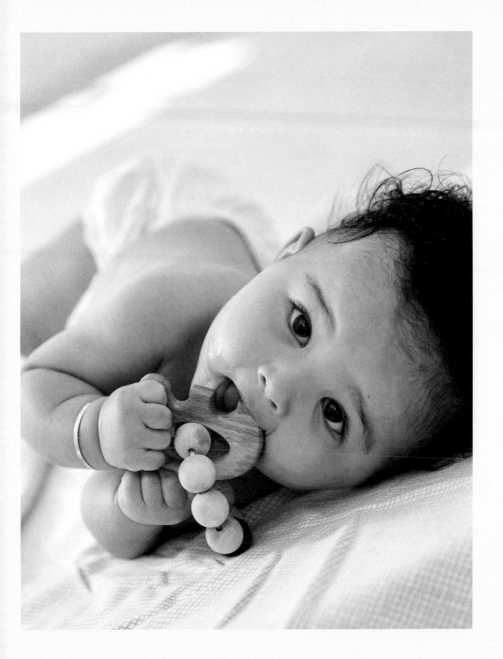

LEGS AND FEET

The legs and feet are a great place to start your exploration of baby massage. Before you begin, pour a small amount of your chosen oil into your hand, and rub your palms together to warm it up.

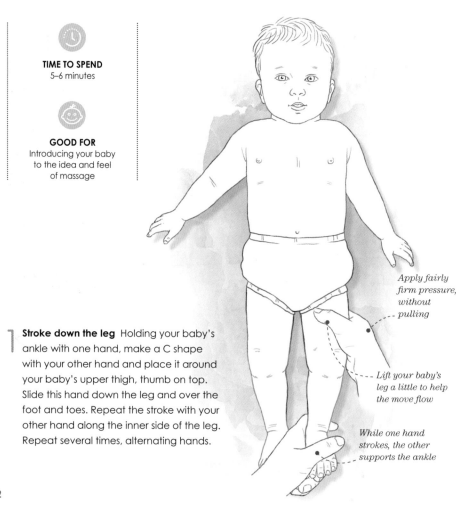

TIME TO SPEND
5–6 minutes

GOOD FOR
Introducing your baby
to the idea and feel
of massage

*Apply fairly
firm pressure,
without
pulling*

1 Stroke down the leg Holding your baby's ankle with one hand, make a C shape with your other hand and place it around your baby's upper thigh, thumb on top. Slide this hand down the leg and over the foot and toes. Repeat the stroke with your other hand along the inner side of the leg. Repeat several times, alternating hands.

*Lift your baby's
leg a little to help
the move flow*

*While one hand
strokes, the other
supports the ankle*

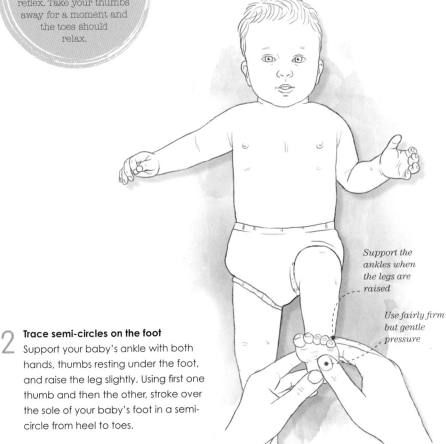

PLANTAR REFLEX
When you touch the sole of your baby's foot the toes will curl, as if gripping, in a natural reflex. Take your thumbs away for a moment and the toes should relax.

Support the ankles when the legs are raised

Use fairly firm but gentle pressure

2 **Trace semi-circles on the foot**
Support your baby's ankle with both hands, thumbs resting under the foot, and raise the leg slightly. Using first one thumb and then the other, stroke over the sole of your baby's foot in a semi-circle from heel to toes.

> *Continued...*   23

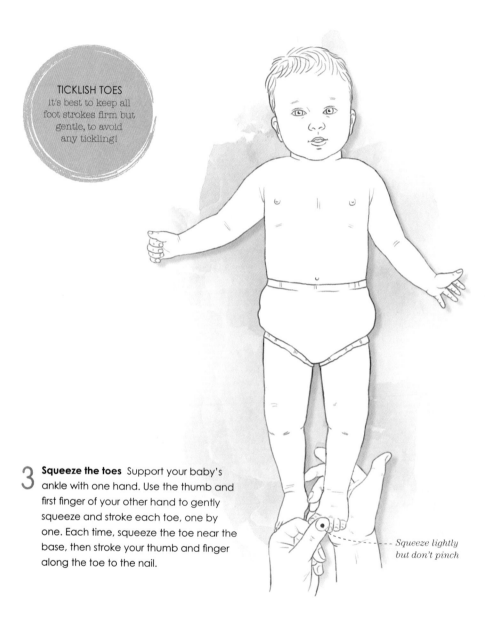

TICKLISH TOES
It's best to keep all foot strokes firm but gentle, to avoid any tickling!

Squeeze lightly but don't pinch

3 **Squeeze the toes** Support your baby's ankle with one hand. Use the thumb and first finger of your other hand to gently squeeze and stroke each toe, one by one. Each time, squeeze the toe near the base, then stroke your thumb and finger along the toe to the nail.

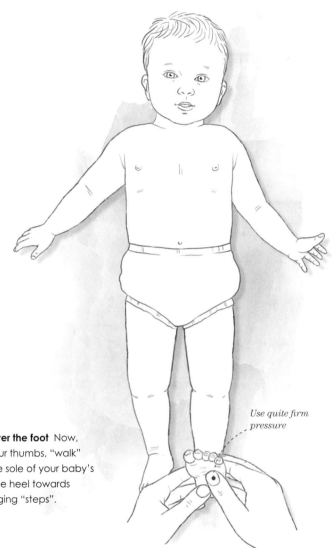

Use quite firm pressure

4 **Walk your thumbs over the foot** Now, using the pads of your thumbs, "walk" your thumbs over the sole of your baby's foot, working from the heel towards the toes in little springing "steps".

≥ *Continued...* 25

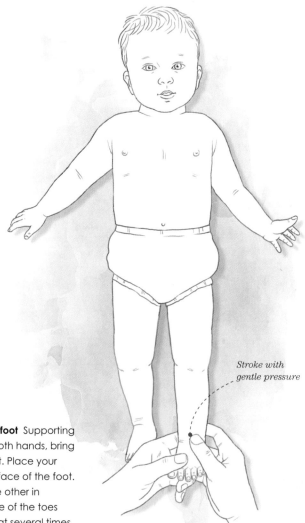

GROWING FEET
These two strokes encourage the bones and muscles of your baby's feet to spread and stretch.

Stroke with gentle pressure

5 **Glide over the top of the foot** Supporting your baby's ankle with both hands, bring their leg down almost flat. Place your thumbs on the upper surface of the foot. Slide one thumb then the other in semi-circles from the base of the toes towards the ankle. Repeat several times.

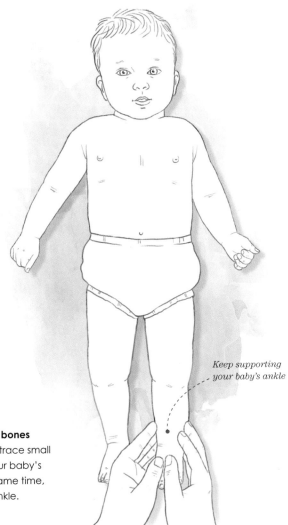

*Keep supporting
your baby's ankle*

6 Make circles around the ankle bones

Use the pads of your fingers to trace small circles around the bones of your baby's ankle. Use both hands at the same time, working on either side of the ankle.

⟩Continued...

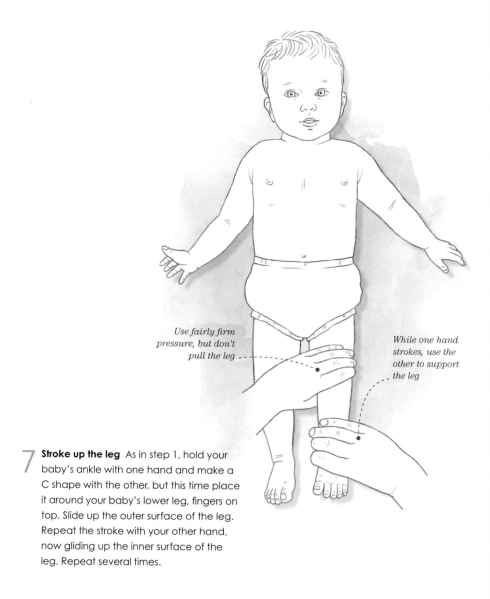

Use fairly firm pressure, but don't pull the leg

While one hand strokes, use the other to support the leg

7 **Stroke up the leg** As in step 1, hold your baby's ankle with one hand and make a C shape with the other, but this time place it around your baby's lower leg, fingers on top. Slide up the outer surface of the leg. Repeat the stroke with your other hand, now gliding up the inner surface of the leg. Repeat several times.

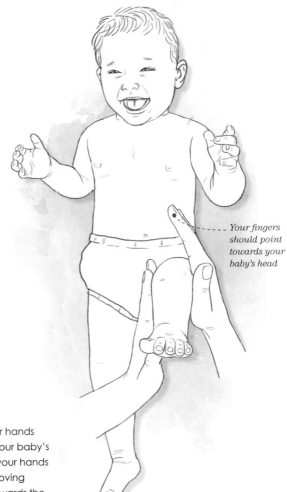

FUN TIME
This stroke is a good one to end on, as it often results in giggles, especially in older babies.

Your fingers should point towards your baby's head

8 **Roll down the leg** Place your hands on either side of the top of your baby's thigh and raise the leg. Roll your hands backwards and forwards, moving down the length of the leg towards the toes. Now repeat steps 1–8 on your baby's other leg.

TUMMY

Babies usually respond well to having their tummy massaged.
By massaging your baby with these strokes, you will be assisting
the natural flow of their digestive system.

TIME TO SPEND
3–4 minutes as part of the
full routine; 8–10 minutes as
a stand-alone massage

GOOD FOR
Smooth digestion

*Relax your
hands and let
them mould to
the shape of your
baby's tummy*

*Don't lift this
hand until your
other hand is
at the top of
the tummy*

Stroke down the tummy Place one hand
horizontally over your baby's tummy, just
under their ribcage, and pause for a
moment. Slide your hand towards the groin,
bringing your other hand to the starting
point on the tummy. Slide that hand over
the tummy too. Repeat 5 or 6 times,
alternating hands in a continuous stroke.

TUMMY TENSION
This stroke is good
for releasing tension
in the abdomen – you
may feel little bubbles
under your thumbs.

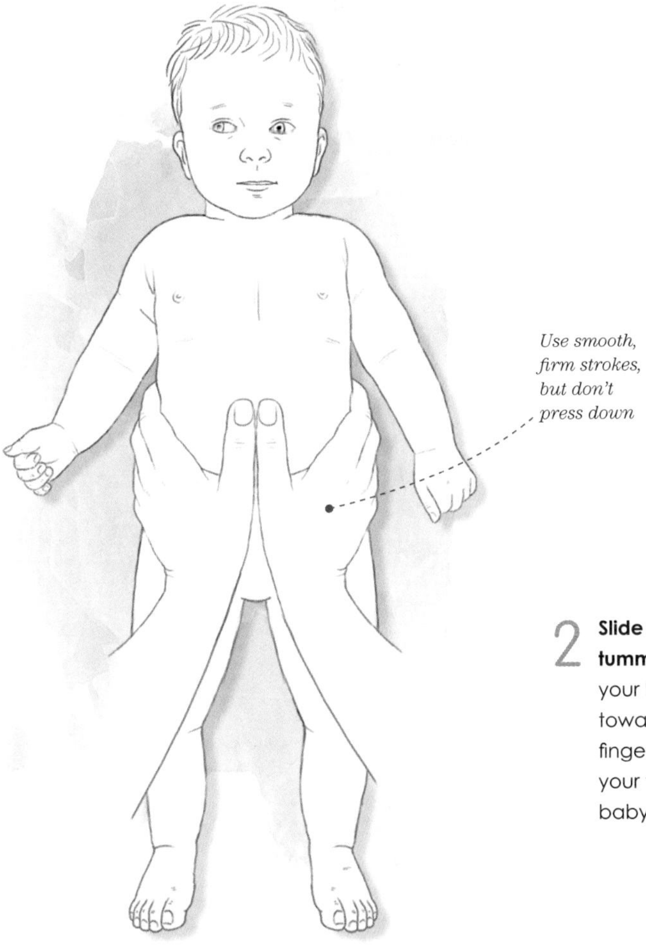

*Use smooth,
firm strokes,
but don't
press down*

2 **Slide your thumbs across the
tummy** Place your thumbs over
your baby's tummy, pointing
towards their head, with your
fingers resting on their waist. Slide
your thumbs out towards your
baby's waist. Repeat 3 or 4 times.

Continued... **31**

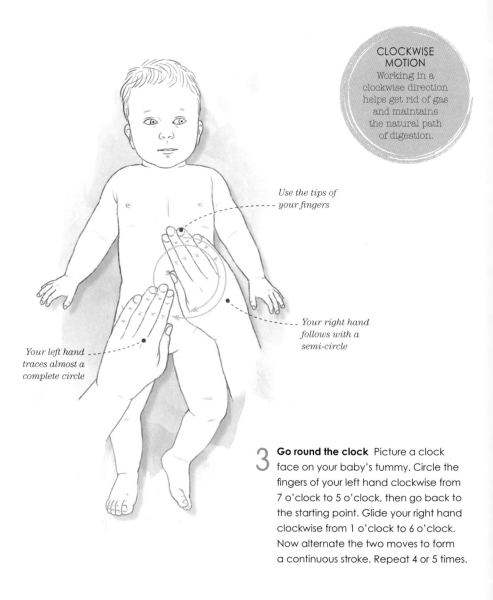

CLOCKWISE
MOTION
Working in a
clockwise direction
helps get rid of gas
and maintains
the natural path
of digestion.

*Use the tips of
your fingers*

*Your right hand
follows with a
semi-circle*

*Your left hand
traces almost a
complete circle*

3 **Go round the clock** Picture a clock
face on your baby's tummy. Circle the
fingers of your left hand clockwise from
7 o'clock to 5 o'clock, then go back to
the starting point. Glide your right hand
clockwise from 1 o'clock to 6 o'clock.
Now alternate the two moves to form
a continuous stroke. Repeat 4 or 5 times.

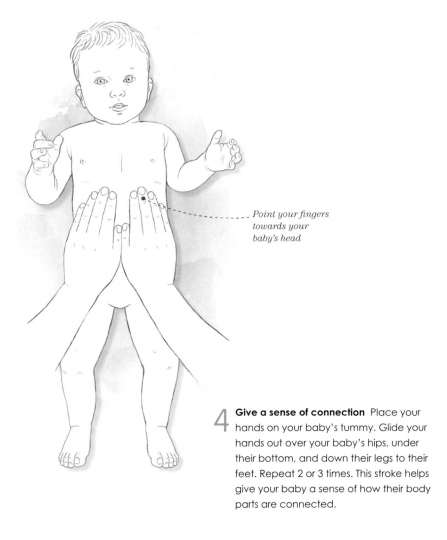

Point your fingers towards your baby's head

4 **Give a sense of connection** Place your hands on your baby's tummy. Glide your hands out over your baby's hips, under their bottom, and down their legs to their feet. Repeat 2 or 3 times. This stroke helps give your baby a sense of how their body parts are connected.

Continued... **33**

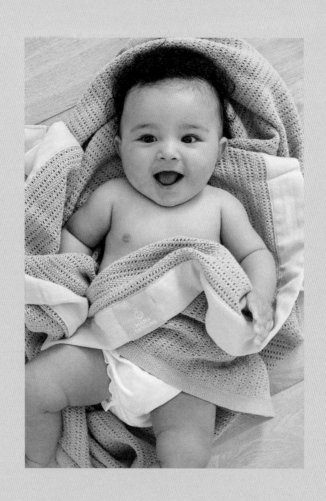

"Regular baby massage enhances the emotional bond between you and your child."

CHEST

Massaging your baby's chest is a lovely way to strengthen your bond: your hands will be over their heart, an area we associate strongly with emotion. If you do not touch this area often, go slowly, but confidently.

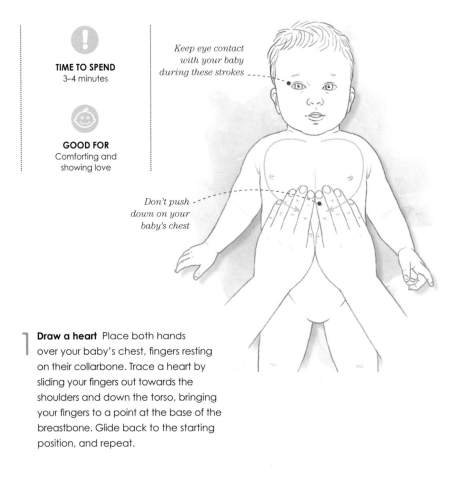

TIME TO SPEND
3–4 minutes

GOOD FOR
Comforting and
showing love

*Keep eye contact
with your baby
during these strokes*

*Don't push
down on your
baby's chest*

1 **Draw a heart** Place both hands over your baby's chest, fingers resting on their collarbone. Trace a heart by sliding your fingers out towards the shoulders and down the torso, bringing your fingers to a point at the base of the breastbone. Glide back to the starting position, and repeat.

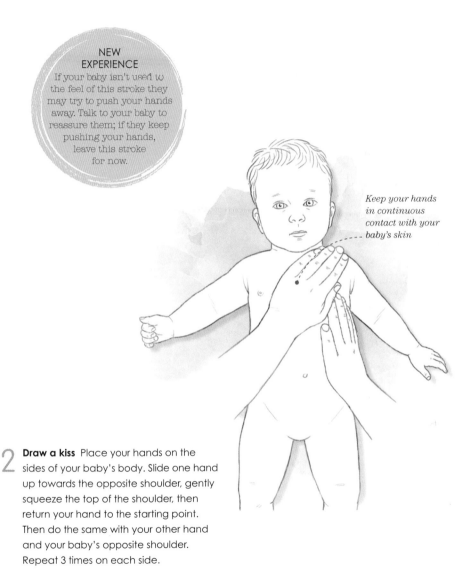

NEW
EXPERIENCE
If your baby isn't used to
the feel of this stroke they
may try to push your hands
away. Talk to your baby to
reassure them; if they keep
pushing your hands,
leave this stroke
for now.

*Keep your hands
in continuous
contact with your
baby's skin*

2 **Draw a kiss** Place your hands on the
sides of your baby's body. Slide one hand
up towards the opposite shoulder, gently
squeeze the top of the shoulder, then
return your hand to the starting point.
Then do the same with your other hand
and your baby's opposite shoulder.
Repeat 3 times on each side.

ARMS AND HANDS

Babies often find it hard to let their arms go floppy. Gently tapping and bouncing your baby's arms will encourage them to relax, as will singing to your baby during the massage.

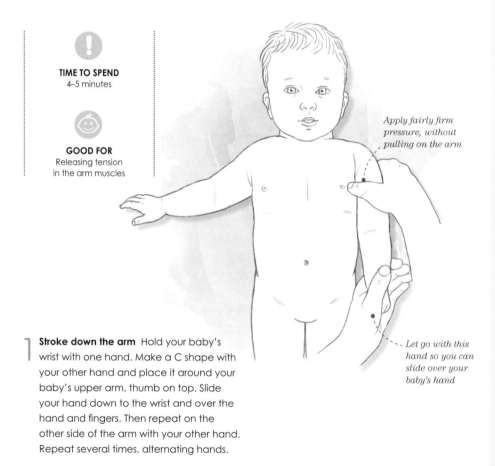

TIME TO SPEND
4–5 minutes

GOOD FOR
Releasing tension in the arm muscles

Apply fairly firm pressure, without pulling on the arm

Let go with this hand so you can slide over your baby's hand

Stroke down the arm Hold your baby's wrist with one hand. Make a C shape with your other hand and place it around your baby's upper arm, thumb on top. Slide your hand down to the wrist and over the hand and fingers. Then repeat on the other side of the arm with your other hand. Repeat several times, alternating hands.

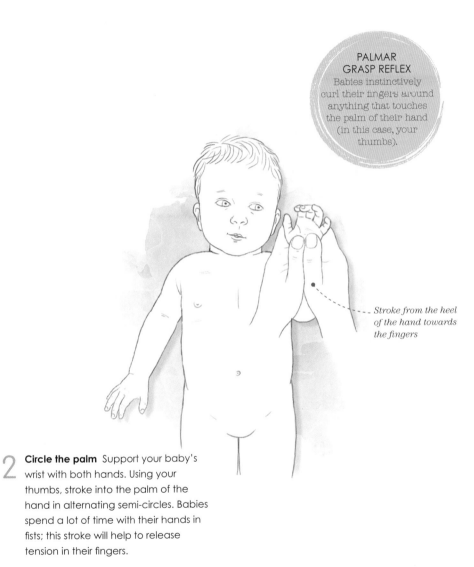

PALMAR
GRASP REFLEX
Babies instinctively
curl their fingers around
anything that touches
the palm of their hand
(in this case, your
thumbs).

*Stroke from the heel
of the hand towards
the fingers*

2 **Circle the palm** Support your baby's
wrist with both hands. Using your
thumbs, stroke into the palm of the
hand in alternating semi-circles. Babies
spend a lot of time with their hands in
fists; this stroke will help to release
tension in their fingers.

>*Continued...* **39**

GETTING COMFY
Your baby may want to hold their arm close to their body during these strokes. Do the massage in a position that is comfortable for you both.

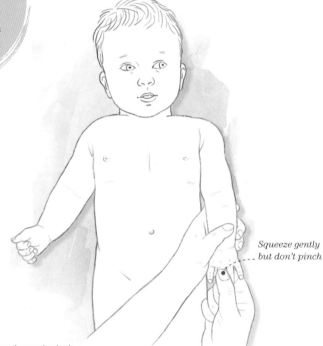

Squeeze gently but don't pinch

3 **Stroke the fingers** Support your baby's wrist with one hand. Use the first and second fingers of your other hand to gently squeeze and stroke each of your baby's fingers, one by one, from the base of each finger to the nail.

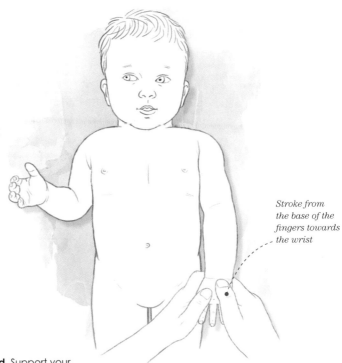

*Stroke from
the base of the
fingers towards
the wrist*

4 **Glide over the hand** Support your
baby's wrist with both hands. Working
on the back of the hand, glide your
thumbs, alternating left and right, in
semi-circles over the back of the hand.

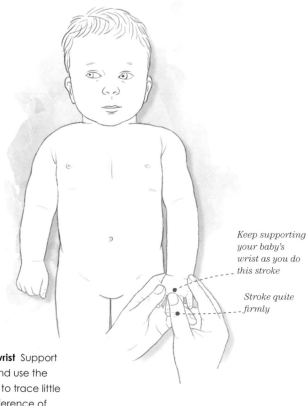

GROWING HANDS
This and the previous stroke support the bones and muscles of your baby's hand and wrist as they grow.

Keep supporting your baby's wrist as you do this stroke

Stroke quite firmly

5 **Make circles around the wrist** Support the arm with one hand, and use the fingers of your other hand to trace little circles around the circumference of your baby's wrist.

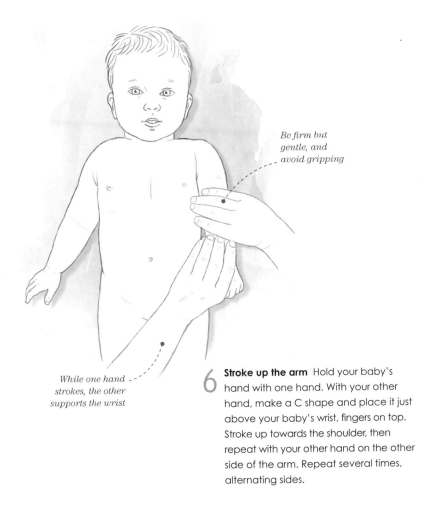

Be firm but gentle, and avoid gripping

While one hand strokes, the other supports the wrist

6 **Stroke up the arm** Hold your baby's hand with one hand. With your other hand, make a C shape and place it just above your baby's wrist, fingers on top. Stroke up towards the shoulder, then repeat with your other hand on the other side of the arm. Repeat several times, alternating sides.

≫ *Continued...*

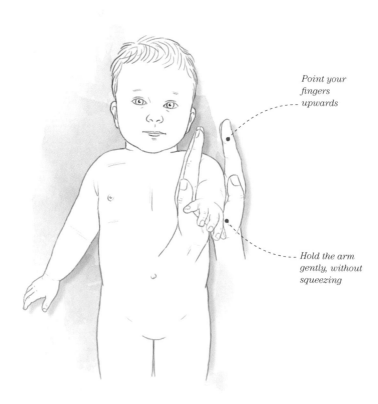

*Point your
fingers
upwards*

*Hold the arm
gently, without
squeezing*

7 **Roll down the arms** Place your hands on either side of the top of your baby's arm. Now roll your hands gently back and forth down the length of the arm towards your baby's hand. Then repeat steps 1–7 on your baby's other arm.

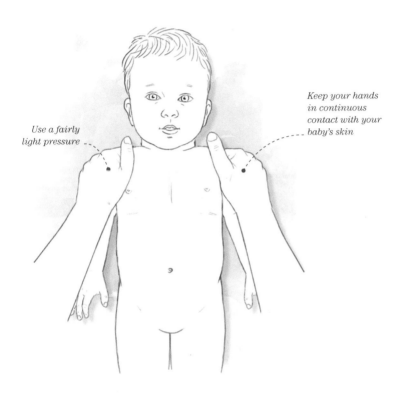

Use a fairly
light pressure

*Keep your hands
in continuous
contact with your
baby's skin*

8 **Finish with a "connection" stroke**
After massaging both arms, finish the
sequence by placing your hands
over your baby's chest. Glide your
hands out over your baby's shoulders
and down their arms to their hands.
Repeat 2 or 3 times.

FACE AND HEAD

Babies don't like a lot of fuss near their face, so be extra gentle when first trying these strokes. Once your baby is used to having their face touched, they will respond with wonderful eye contact and a state of relaxation.

TIME TO SPEND
2–3 minutes

GOOD FOR
Helping with a stuffy nose or teething pain, and relaxing the muscles of the face

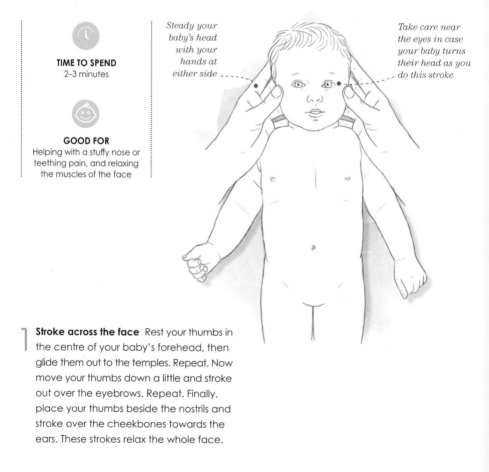

Steady your baby's head with your hands at either side

Take care near the eyes in case your baby turns their head as you do this stroke

1 **Stroke across the face** Rest your thumbs in the centre of your baby's forehead, then glide them out to the temples. Repeat. Now move your thumbs down a little and stroke out over the eyebrows. Repeat. Finally, place your thumbs beside the nostrils and stroke over the cheekbones towards the ears. These strokes relax the whole face.

CONGESTION
The first step in this sequence is particularly useful if your baby is snuffly, as it helps drain the sinuses – see page 100.

Use fairly firm pressure

2 **Make circles over the cheeks** Rest your hands on your baby's chest, and use the pads of your fingers to make gentle circular strokes over your baby's cheeks. This stroke relaxes the hard-working cheek muscles, which can become tired from all that feeding!

Continued...

ROOTING
Babies under 4 months will open their mouth when you touch the lower half of their face – this is called the rooting reflex.

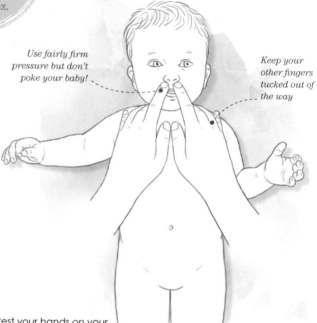

Use fairly firm pressure but don't poke your baby!

Keep your other fingers tucked out of the way

3 **Make a smile** Rest your hands on your baby's chest with your index fingers just above the centre of their top lip. Use both fingers at the same time to stroke out along the top lip. Repeat the stroke just under the lower lip. You should be stroking the skin above and below the lips rather than the lips themselves.

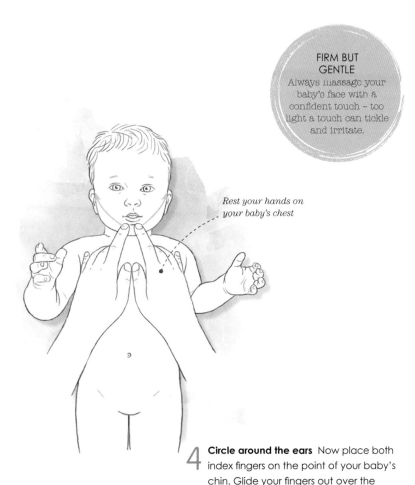

FIRM BUT GENTLE
Always massage your baby's face with a confident touch – too light a touch can tickle and irritate.

Rest your hands on your baby's chest

4 **Circle around the ears** Now place both index fingers on the point of your baby's chin. Glide your fingers out over the cheeks to the tops of the ears, then around and behind the ears, and back to the starting point. This stroke relaxes the lower half of your baby's face and soothes the pain of teething (see page 94).

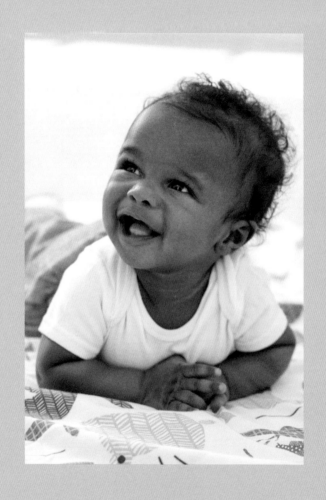

" Research points to the positive effects of communicating through touch; it makes babies feel loved and secure. "

BACK

To massage your baby's back you will need to turn them over onto their front. Babies who can support their neck should be comfortable in this position; very young babies may only be happy for a couple of minutes.

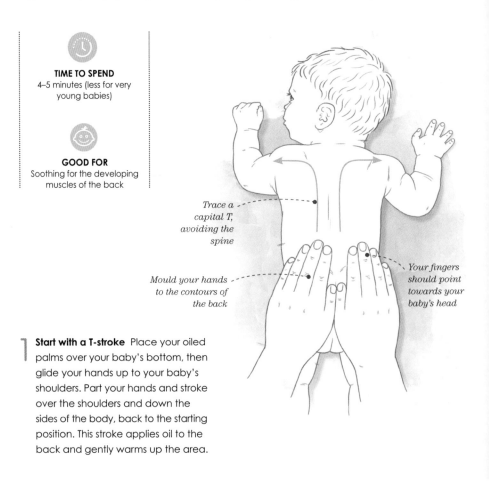

TIME TO SPEND
4–5 minutes (less for very young babies)

GOOD FOR
Soothing for the developing muscles of the back

Trace a capital T, avoiding the spine

Mould your hands to the contours of the back

Your fingers should point towards your baby's head

1 **Start with a T-stroke** Place your oiled palms over your baby's bottom, then glide your hands up to your baby's shoulders. Part your hands and stroke over the shoulders and down the sides of the body, back to the starting position. This stroke applies oil to the back and gently warms up the area.

ON THE MOVE
This stroke will relax the muscles to support movement – great for babies getting ready to crawl.

Keep your hands relaxed

Move your hands in opposite directions

2 **Stroke side to side across the back** To work a little deeper into the muscles, place your hands horizontally over your baby's lower back, then glide them from side to side. Move up and down the body several times repeating this stroke.

> *Continued...*

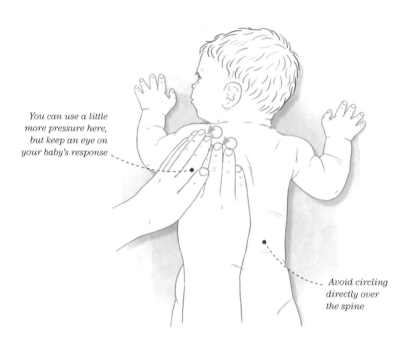

You can use a little more pressure here, but keep an eye on your baby's response

Avoid circling directly over the spine

3 **Make small circles** Place both hands at one side of your baby's spine near their shoulder (you may need to overlap your hands). Using just the pads of your fingers, make small circles over that half of the back, working down towards your baby's bottom. Repeat on the other side.

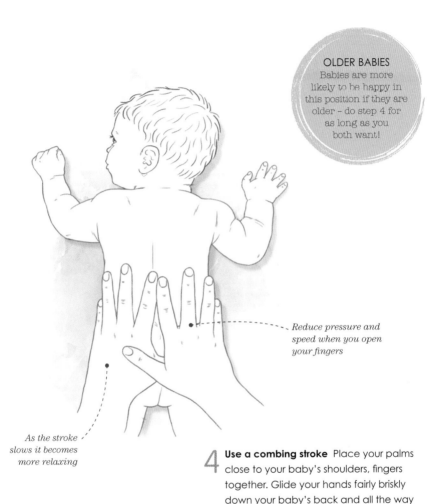

OLDER BABIES
Babies are more likely to be happy in this position if they are older – do step 4 for as long as you both want!

Reduce pressure and speed when you open your fingers

As the stroke slows it becomes more relaxing

4 **Use a combing stroke** Place your palms close to your baby's shoulders, fingers together. Glide your hands fairly briskly down your baby's back and all the way to their ankles, then repeat. Now open your fingers and slow the stroke down. Repeat a few times, gradually coming to a stop. Finish the massage with a cuddle.

YOUR DAILY ROUTINE

YOUR DAILY ROUTINE

In this chapter you'll find massage sequences for specific moments in your baby's day, ready for you to incorporate into your own routine at the times that suit you best.

FINDING THE RIGHT TIME

You are the best judge of when your baby is most receptive to massage. The most important thing is finding a time that works for you and your baby; once you do, massage can become something to look forward to every day.

EVERYDAY CARE

At playtime, have fun with yoga-like stretches. Babies tend to be very flexible – these moves will encourage that flexibility and support muscle growth, as well as stimulating your baby's nervous system and helping them to become more aware of their body. Fun for both of you, playtime is the perfect chance to relax, sing songs, and make your baby laugh.

Nappy changing is often a convenient time to tack on a quick massage. The short routine on page 66 is quick enough to fit into a busy day, but still effective at soothing your baby and communicating love.

There are also some strokes here that are suitable for using in an even quicker massage session while on the go. In the face of stressful situations, when you can't easily take your baby off to a quiet location and perform a full massage, even just a little soothing touch can work wonders at calming your baby – and you – down.

Last but not least comes a massage routine for the end of the day. It is worth bearing in mind that even though a massage before bed might be an appealing idea from your perspective, if your baby is already settling down it may not be worth the risk of stimulating them too much. Leave time for a massage then a feed before putting your baby to bed, and stick to your routine once it's established.

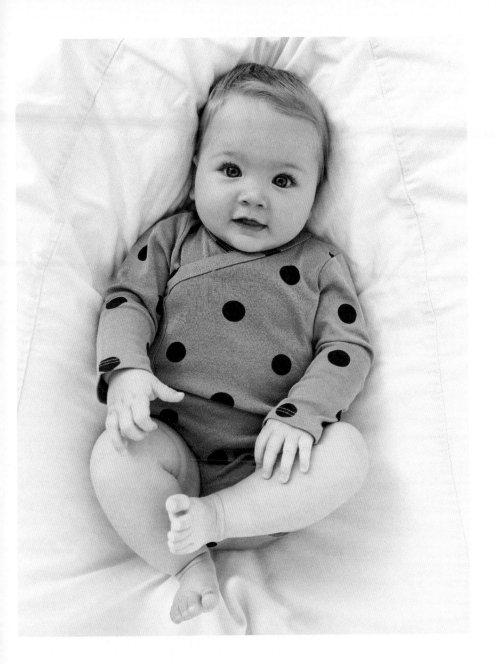

PLAYTIME

This playful, stimulating routine is for fun rather than relaxation, and may even make your baby giggle! These moves will also support growth, aid flexibility, and help your baby become more aware of their own body.

MASSAGE AS PLAY

This routine is suitable for babies of around 6 months and older. It's more physical than the other routines in this book, and is best left for a time when you feel your baby needs some attention that is stimulating and playful – the last move in particular often makes babies laugh, especially older babies. There is no upper age limit with this sequence; you can adapt the strokes as your baby grows.

The floor is the best place to do this routine; get comfy and have fun! Your baby can be dressed or not, and there is no need to use oil for this sequence. It's a good idea to talk or even sing as you practise these moves – see if you can recall nursery rhymes that you may have known as a child, or just sing whatever you like!

FINDING THE RIGHT TIME

Don't be tempted to practise this routine if your baby is due a feed or a nap – the result will be a cranky baby and a disappointed parent. Find a time in their day when you know they will respond to some stimulation: during the afternoon may be a good opportunity, when you have time to interact and play. Spend at least 10 minutes on the routine, or longer if you and your baby are happy to continue.

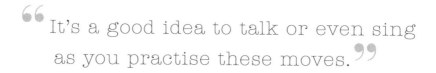

“ It's a good idea to talk or even sing as you practise these moves. ”

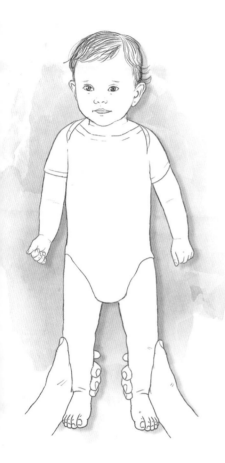

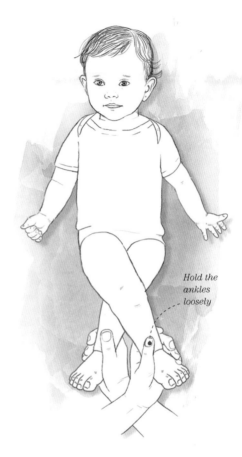

Hold the ankles loosely

1 **Bounce the legs** Lay your baby on their back. Support each of your baby's ankles in your hands and gently bounce their legs.

2 **Cross the legs** Still supporting your baby's ankles, gently cross their legs one way then the other. Gently stretch your baby's legs out straight. Repeat 5 or 6 times. Do not take your baby's legs out to the sides.

> *Continued...*

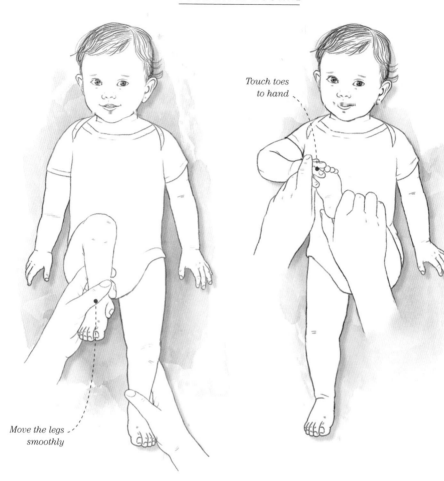

Touch toes to hand

Move the legs smoothly

3 **Cycle the legs** Hold your baby's ankles, one in each hand. Gently cycle their legs towards their tummy. Then reverse the direction of the cycling and bring the legs back down flat. Tell your baby what you are doing: "cycling up the hill, cycling down the hill" – make it a game!

4 **Stretch opposite limbs** Hold one of your baby's ankles in one hand, and their opposite wrist in the other. Bring ankle and wrist together. Then gently stretch the arm above the head and lower the leg flat. Repeat 3 or 4 times, then do the same with the other arm and leg.

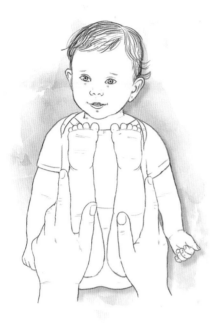

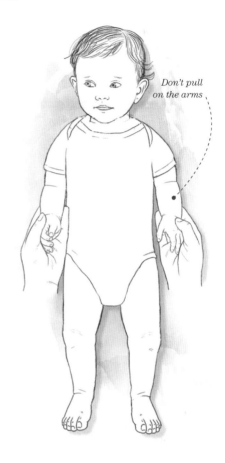

Don't pull on the arms

5 **Bring toes to nose** Take hold of your baby's legs and gently lift their toes towards their face. Many babies spontaneously bring their toes up to their mouth to investigate them; this move encourages your baby to explore their body. Stop pushing if you feel resistance.

6 **Bounce the arms** Hold onto your baby's hands or wrists and gently bounce their arms. This is a great move to encourage your baby to relax their arms, which commonly hold tension.

❯ *Continued...*

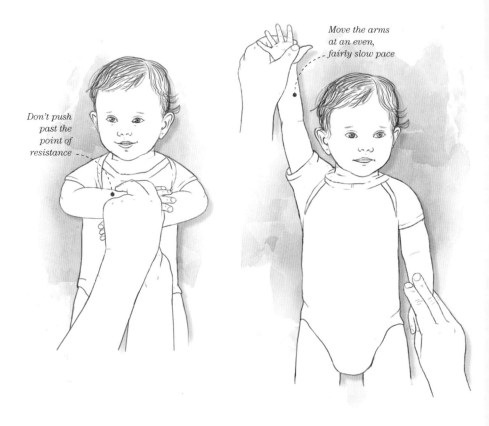

Don't push past the point of resistance - - -

Move the arms at an even, fairly slow pace - -

7 **Cross the arms** Hold onto your baby's hands or wrists, one in each hand. Gently cross the arms over the chest, first one way, then the other. Then gently stretch the arms out to the sides, away from the body. Repeat 5 or 6 times. If your baby isn't enjoying this move, repeat step 6 instead.

8 **March the arms** Hold onto your baby's hands or wrists, one in each hand. Gently march their arms up and down, one arm above the head, one arm down the body, and so on, for about a minute.

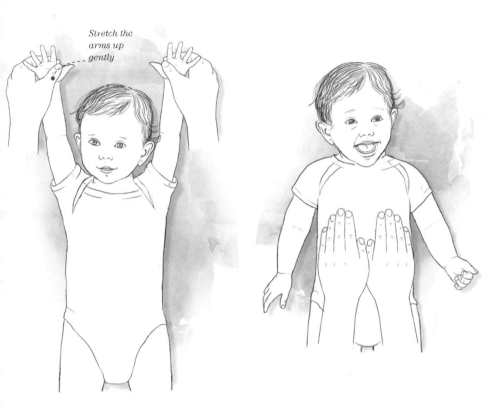

Stretch the arms up gently

9 **Reach high and stretch low** Use both hands to hold onto your baby's hands or wrists. Gently stretch both of their arms up over their head. Then bring their arms back down to the starting position.

10 **Stroke from top to toes** With both hands, stroke from the top of your baby's head right down to their toes, over their whole body. This stroke gives your baby a real sense of being all joined up. Repeat several times, then finish with a cuddle!

NAPPY TIME

Right after changing your baby's nappy is the perfect time to fit in a short massage routine. Even just a few extra moments of close contact during the day will strengthen your bond with your baby.

A CHANCE TO BOND

Changing nappies might not be the most enjoyable part of caring for a baby, but a nappy change can be a great chance to spend some time in close contact with your little one, as well as an opportunity to sneak in a quick massage during a busy day. Babies often enjoy the chance to kick their legs about without their nappy on – make the most of this time with some comforting massage strokes too. This short routine is also ideal for relaxing your baby before a daytime nap.

THE RIGHT MOOD

This is a convenient time for a massage as your baby is already half-undressed. If you're in a hurry, or your baby is fractious, put the massage off until later. If your baby is happy, though, try this short sequence.

Have everything to hand before you begin: your chosen vegetable oil, a spare towel, and wipes. Do these strokes after cleaning your baby, but before putting on a fresh nappy. Pour a small amount of oil into the palm of your hand then rub your hands together to warm them up, before you begin.

66 A nappy change can be a chance to spend some time in close contact with your little one. 99

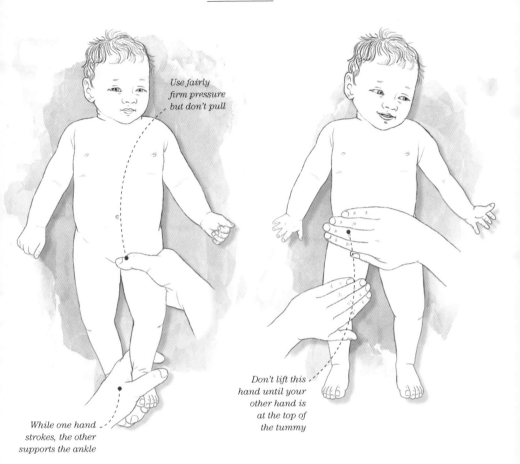

Use fairly firm pressure but don't pull

While one hand strokes, the other supports the ankle

Don't lift this hand until your other hand is at the top of the tummy

1 **Stroke along the legs** Make a C shape with your hand and place it around your baby's upper thigh, thumb on top. Stroke down the leg and over the foot. Then stroke down the other side of the leg with your other hand. Repeat. Now change direction, starting at the ankle, fingers on top, and gliding up. Repeat several times on both legs.

2 **Stroke down the tummy** Place one hand horizontally at the top of your baby's tummy and pause for a moment. Slide your hand down towards your baby's groin, bringing your other hand to the starting point on the tummy. Alternating hands, stroke continuously over the tummy 5 or 6 times.

≻*Continued...*   **67**

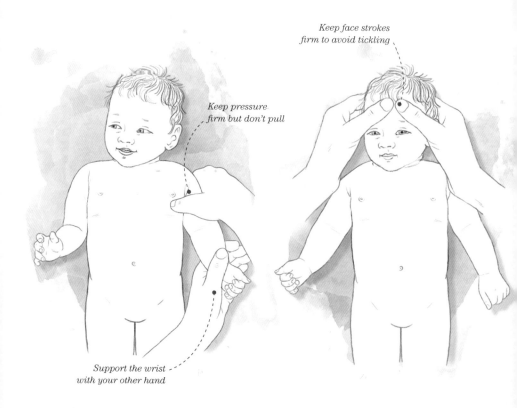

*Keep face strokes
firm to avoid tickling*

*Keep pressure
firm but don't pull*

*Support the wrist
with your other hand*

3 **Stroke along the arms** Make a C shape with your hand. Place it around your baby's upper arm, thumb on top. Stroke down the arm and over the hand. Then stroke down the other side of the arm with your other hand. Repeat, then change direction, starting at the wrist, thumb underneath. Repeat several times on both arms.

4 **Stroke the forehead** Place your hands at either side of your baby's head, with your thumbs resting in the centre of their forehead. Glide your thumbs from the centre of the forehead out to the temples. Repeat.

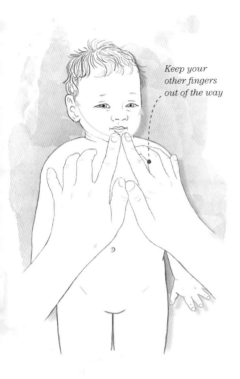

Keep your
other fingers
out of the way

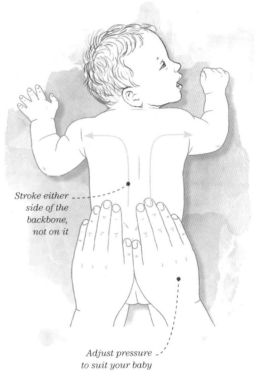

Stroke either
side of the
backbone,
not on it

Adjust pressure
to suit your baby

5 **Stroke around the ears** Now bring your hands to rest on your baby's chest, with the first finger of each hand on the point of your baby's chin. Glide both fingers out over the cheeks, towards the tops of the ears, around and behind the ears, then back to the starting point.

6 **Do a T-stroke on the back** Turn your baby onto their front, then place your hands over their bottom. Glide your hands gently but firmly up your baby's back. Part your hands at the shoulders, then stroke over them and down the sides of the body back to your starting position. Repeat several times, then finish the massage with a cuddle.

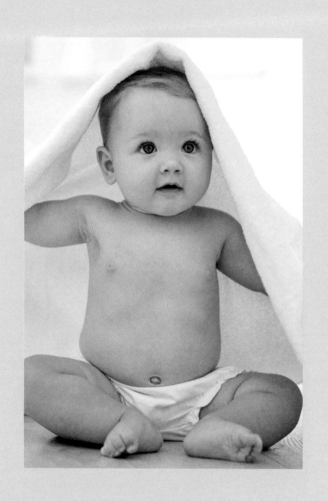

"Babies respond very well to a soft, sing-song tone – talk or sing during a massage to boost bonding."

OUT AND ABOUT

Ideally a massage should be carried out at home, in a relaxed atmosphere and with little or no interruptions. Sometimes, though, it is while out and about that you need a quick way to comfort and soothe your little one.

MASSAGE ON THE MOVE

We've all been stuck in traffic, waiting in a queue, or desperate to arrive at our destination... all of these things may make you and your baby feel frustrated. Taking a few deep breaths and performing some simple massage techniques may go some way to soothing your baby and returning home relatively unscathed. These strokes are best done without oil and can be done through clothing. It is possible to perform them while your baby is strapped into their pushchair, car seat, or carrier; just adapt the strokes slightly to focus on the areas of your baby that you're able to reach.

A REASSURING ROUTINE

Babies respond well to repetition; it helps them learn and makes them feel secure. If while out and about you are confronted with a stressful situation for you and your baby, making use of massage techniques can help to calm things down. A baby who is massaged regularly will learn to relax at your soft touch and words of reassurance.

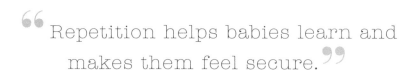

“Repetition helps babies learn and makes them feel secure.”

Relax your hand

Stroke your baby With firm but gentle pressure, stroke whatever part of your baby you can reach in your current situation. Speak with a soothing voice as you repeat the move, encouraging your baby to relax.

>*Continued...* **73**

COMFORTING
WORDS
Talk to your baby all
the while, keeping
what you say simple
and repetitive.

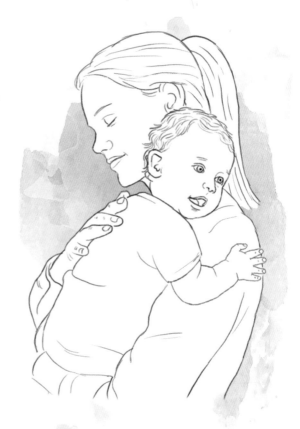

2 **Gently pat your baby** With an open
palm, gently tap over the areas of your
baby's body that you can reach. This
move works particularly well over the
back, as it's a comparatively large area;
a soft, rhythmic tapping over the back
can soothe and comfort your baby.

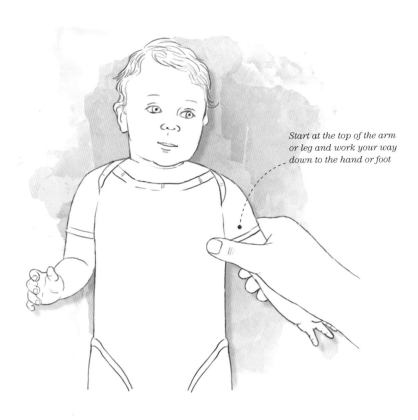

Start at the top of the arm or leg and work your way down to the hand or foot

3 **Gently squeeze your baby's arms or legs**
With one hand, gently squeeze down your baby's arms or legs. Squeeze lightly, release, and move your hand down slightly, then squeeze again, and so on.

BEDTIME

A massage at bedtime can be a loving way to help your baby settle and sleep – a goal for all parents. This short sequence is easy to incorporate into your bedtime routine, and is ideal for helping your baby relax and drift off.

THE IMPORTANCE OF SLEEP

Babies need sleep to grow and develop. Newborn babies will only sleep between three and five hours at night, but by four months most babies will sleep for longer stretches; up to eight or nine hours in some cases. Sleeping through the night often takes time, though, and getting your baby to settle down and sleep at night can feel like a battle.

While there is no guarantee that massage will always work, it is one way to help your baby wind down before bedtime, and can get them to drift off to sleep. This sequence of strokes can encourage your baby to relax their muscles and close their eyes. However, there are many reasons why babies don't settle; if you are concerned about your baby's sleeping pattern speak to your health visitor or GP.

YOUR BABY'S ROUTINE

To fit in a massage before bed, you will need to bring your usual bedtime routine forward by half an hour or more, so that your baby is not over-tired and fractious. Create a routine that you'll be able to repeat every evening: for instance, you may wish to do a massage after your baby's evening bath. It is best to do the massage before the last feed of the day.

BEFORE YOU BEGIN

If you are using oil, have this along with towels or wipes to hand before you start; you can also do these strokes over your baby's pyjamas or sleepsuit. Do the massage where your baby will be sleeping. Switch off bright lights, make sure the room is warm, and keep stimulation to a minimum. You may wish to play some gentle music, or even sing softly. Lay your baby on their back, then proceed with the following strokes.

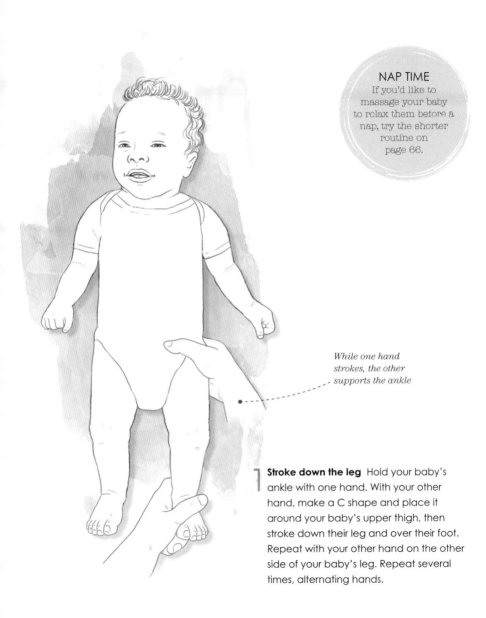

NAP TIME
If you'd like to massage your baby to relax them before a nap, try the shorter routine on page 66.

While one hand strokes, the other supports the ankle

Stroke down the leg Hold your baby's ankle with one hand. With your other hand, make a C shape and place it around your baby's upper thigh, then stroke down their leg and over their foot. Repeat with your other hand on the other side of your baby's leg. Repeat several times, alternating hands.

> *Continued...*   **77**

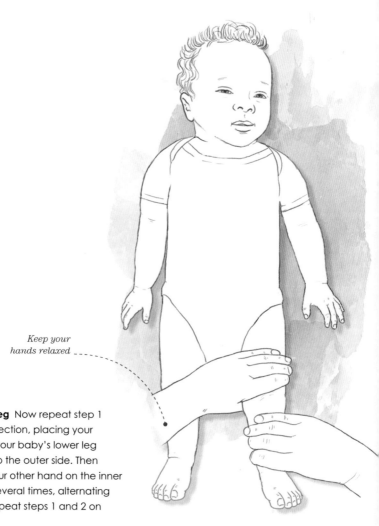

Keep your hands relaxed

2 **Stroke up the leg** Now repeat step 1 in the other direction, placing your hand around your baby's lower leg and stroking up the outer side. Then repeat with your other hand on the inner side. Repeat several times, alternating hands. Then repeat steps 1 and 2 on the other leg.

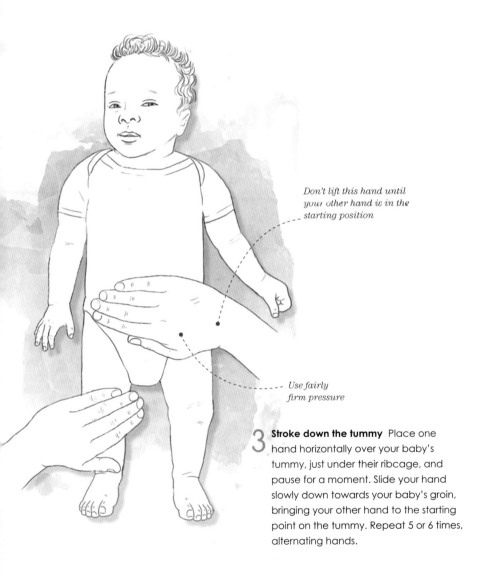

Don't lift this hand until your other hand is in the starting position

Use fairly firm pressure

3 Stroke down the tummy Place one hand horizontally over your baby's tummy, just under their ribcage, and pause for a moment. Slide your hand slowly down towards your baby's groin, bringing your other hand to the starting point on the tummy. Repeat 5 or 6 times, alternating hands.

Continued... **79**

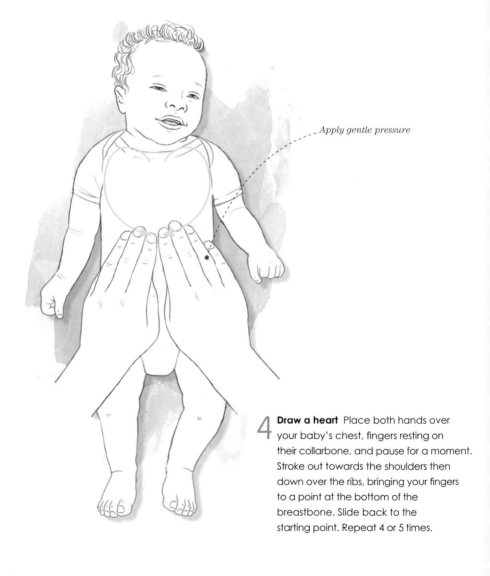

Apply gentle pressure

4 **Draw a heart** Place both hands over your baby's chest, fingers resting on their collarbone, and pause for a moment. Stroke out towards the shoulders then down over the ribs, bringing your fingers to a point at the bottom of the breastbone. Slide back to the starting point. Repeat 4 or 5 times.

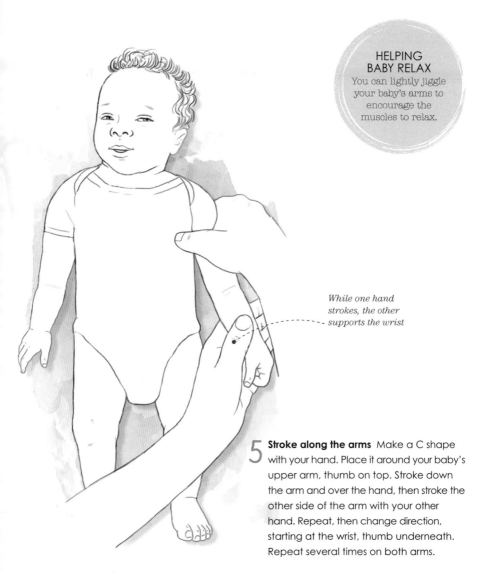

HELPING BABY RELAX
You can lightly jiggle your baby's arms to encourage the muscles to relax.

While one hand strokes, the other supports the wrist

5 **Stroke along the arms** Make a C shape with your hand. Place it around your baby's upper arm, thumb on top. Stroke down the arm and over the hand, then stroke the other side of the arm with your other hand. Repeat, then change direction, starting at the wrist, thumb underneath. Repeat several times on both arms.

❯ *Continued...* **81**

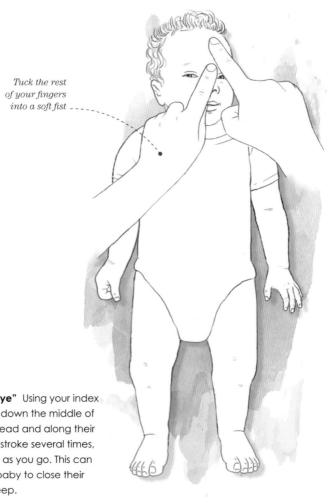

Tuck the rest of your fingers into a soft fist

6 **Stroke the "third eye"** Using your index finger only, stroke down the middle of your baby's forehead and along their nose. Repeat the stroke several times, alternating hands as you go. This can encourage your baby to close their eyes, ready for sleep.

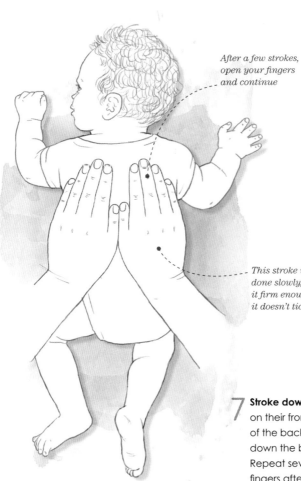

After a few strokes, open your fingers and continue

This stroke is best done slowly, but keep it firm enough so that it doesn't tickle

7 **Stroke down the back** Place your baby on their front. Place your hands at the top of the back, either side of the spine. Glide down the back and legs to the ankles. Repeat several times, opening your fingers after a few strokes. Slow down, then stop. Cuddle your baby, then either lay them down to sleep or feed them.

EASING COMMON AILMENTS

EASING COMMON AILMENTS

In this chapter you'll find routines to address some common baby ailments – for these issues, massage can be just the thing to get your baby feeling well again.

HEALING TOUCH

When babies are feeling off-colour, they can often be comforted by a loving, soothing touch, especially when it's combined with vocal reassurances. Massage can help in two ways: it calms your baby down, and it can lessen symptoms, by giving the immune system a boost, improving circulation, and encouraging waste to move out of the body, all of which help your baby fight illness and feel better.

Here you'll find routines to help with some of the minor upsets that many babies experience – teething, congestion, colic, and constipation – as well as advice on massaging babies with skin concerns.

MASSAGE FOR MINOR AILMENTS

The routines in this chapter are short and targeted to particular concerns. You can do any of them as a stand-alone treatment, or incorporate them into your routine until your baby is feeling happy and healthy again.

Keep in mind that while massage has proven health benefits, it is not a substitute for necessary medical care. It is very important to speak to your baby's doctor or health visitor if you have any concerns about your baby's health. Don't massage your baby if they have an upset tummy or a temperature – these are situations when you should consult a medical professional.

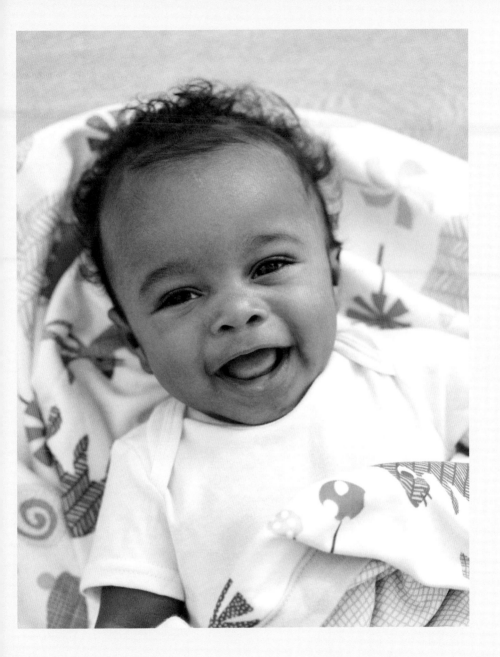

COLIC AND CONSTIPATION

Colic – when gas gets trapped in your baby's digestive system – and constipation often cause discomfort. It's hard to soothe a baby when they are in pain, but tummy massage can lessen the symptoms.

RELIEVING COLIC

If your baby has colic their tummy might become quite firm and they may squirm with discomfort. They may also bring their legs up to their tummy or arch their backs. While there is no guarantee that massage will banish your baby's colic, it can provide temporary relief by encouraging movement in the digestive system, which helps your baby expel wind.

Colic often seems to be worse in the early evening. Try doing this massage sequence before your baby's "regular" upset time, and you may be able to prevent the symptoms. If your baby gets upset, take a deep breath and keep going for a little while to see if you can soothe their tummy – if they don't settle, stop and try again another time. Colic should pass altogether when your baby reaches approximately 6 months of age.

RELIEVING CONSTIPATION

Another common problem for babies and children is constipation. Massaging the abdomen in a clockwise circular motion can help to get things moving, encouraging digested food to pass through your baby's gut; gently bending and bouncing their legs can help to open their bowels. In addition to massage, make sure your baby is drinking enough fluids and eating a balanced diet if they have been weaned.

WHEN TO USE THIS SEQUENCE

It's fine to do this routine without oil and through clothing, if needed, though as with all massage it will be more beneficial if your baby is naked. Always wait for at least an hour after a feed before performing this sequence. While these strokes can bring relief from colic, constipation, and excessive wind, don't massage your baby if they have an upset tummy or diarrhoea. Always check with your health visitor or GP if you have any concerns about your baby's wellbeing.

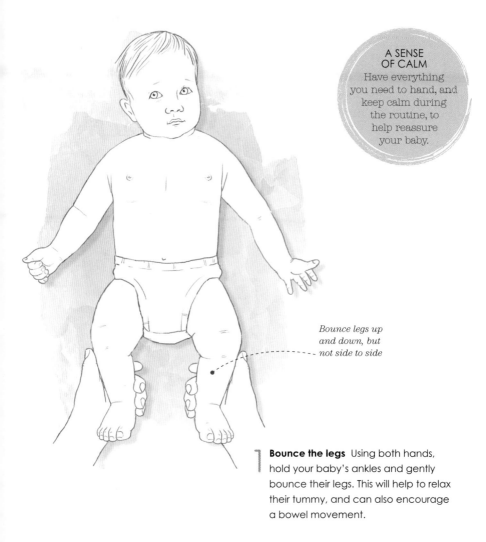

A SENSE
OF CALM
Have everything
you need to hand, and
keep calm during
the routine, to
help reassure
your baby.

*Bounce legs up
and down, but
not side to side*

Bounce the legs Using both hands,
hold your baby's ankles and gently
bounce their legs. This will help to relax
their tummy, and can also encourage
a bowel movement.

> *Continued...* **89**

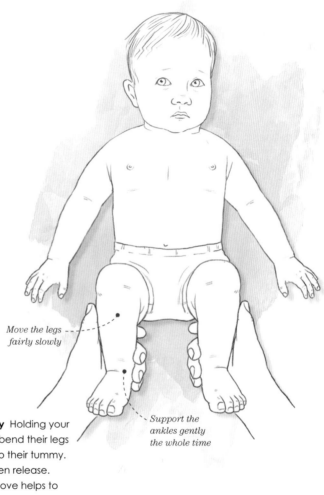

*Move the legs
fairly slowly*

*Support the
ankles gently
the whole time*

2 **Push knees into tummy** Holding your
baby's ankles, gently bend their legs
to push their knees into their tummy.
Hold for 5 seconds, then release.
Repeat 3 times. This move helps to
ease pain caused by trapped wind.

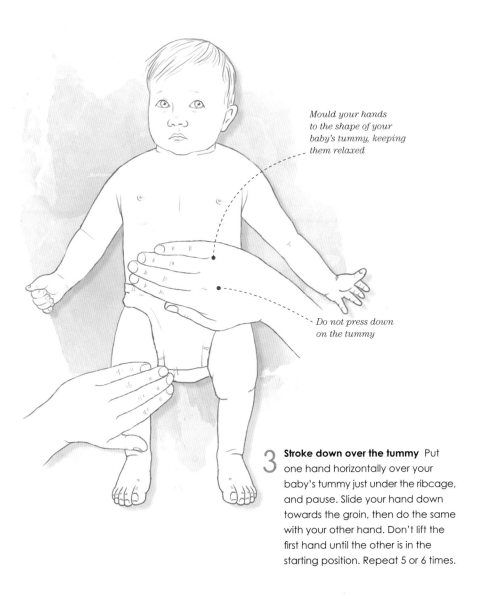

*Mould your hands
to the shape of your
baby's tummy, keeping
them relaxed*

*Do not press down
on the tummy*

3 Stroke down over the tummy Put one hand horizontally over your baby's tummy just under the ribcage, and pause. Slide your hand down towards the groin, then do the same with your other hand. Don't lift the first hand until the other is in the starting position. Repeat 5 or 6 times.

▶ *Continued...* **91**

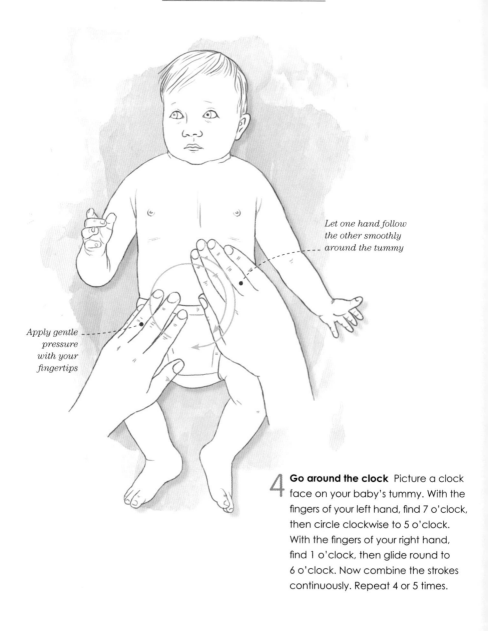

Let one hand follow the other smoothly around the tummy

Apply gentle pressure with your fingertips

4 **Go around the clock** Picture a clock face on your baby's tummy. With the fingers of your left hand, find 7 o'clock, then circle clockwise to 5 o'clock. With the fingers of your right hand, find 1 o'clock, then glide round to 6 o'clock. Now combine the strokes continuously. Repeat 4 or 5 times.

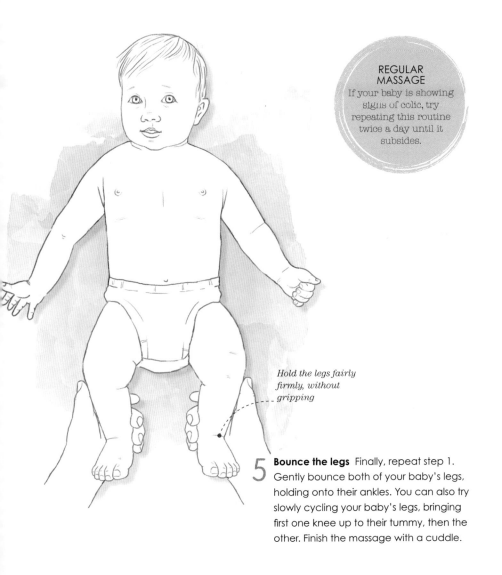

REGULAR MASSAGE
If your baby is showing signs of colic, try repeating this routine twice a day until it subsides.

Hold the legs fairly firmly, without gripping

5 **Bounce the legs** Finally, repeat step 1. Gently bounce both of your baby's legs, holding onto their ankles. You can also try slowly cycling your baby's legs, bringing first one knee up to their tummy, then the other. Finish the massage with a cuddle.

TEETHING

When your baby starts teething, their sore gums can be a cause of upset for both of you. Gentle massage strokes over the face and jaw are a great way to help soothe the pain.

TEETHING TROUBLES

All babies have a different reaction to teething. Some babies are even born with teeth! On average, though, teeth start to emerge at around 4–6 months. By the time your baby is two years old they will have most of their baby teeth.

If your baby is teething, they may have reddened cheeks and may pull at their ears as if they are uncomfortable. They may have a raised temperature and will probably dribble a lot and want to chew. Sometimes teething seems to result in a tummy upset and an increase in nappy rash, though there is no medical evidence to support this.

SOOTHING SORE GUMS

To temporarily ease the pain of teething, try massaging your baby's face around their gums and jaw using the following sequence of strokes. This will encourage the muscles of your baby's face to relax, boost blood flow around the mouth – which will speed up the teething process – and counteract the pressure of the new teeth below the gums.

66 To ease the pain of teething, try massaging your baby's face around their gums and jaw. 99

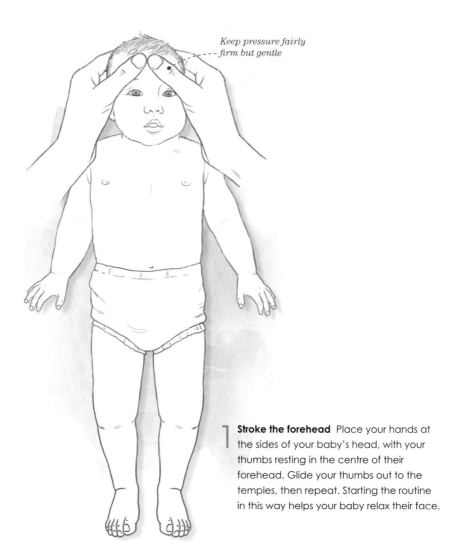

Keep pressure fairly firm but gentle

Stroke the forehead Place your hands at the sides of your baby's head, with your thumbs resting in the centre of their forehead. Glide your thumbs out to the temples, then repeat. Starting the routine in this way helps your baby relax their face.

⟩ *Continued...* **95**

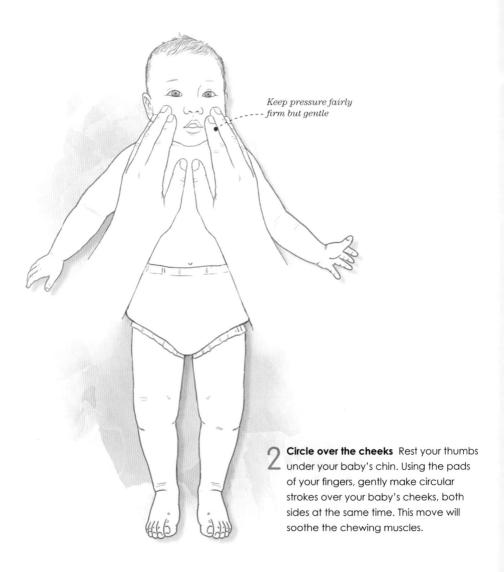

Keep pressure fairly firm but gentle

2 **Circle over the cheeks** Rest your thumbs under your baby's chin. Using the pads of your fingers, gently make circular strokes over your baby's cheeks, both sides at the same time. This move will soothe the chewing muscles.

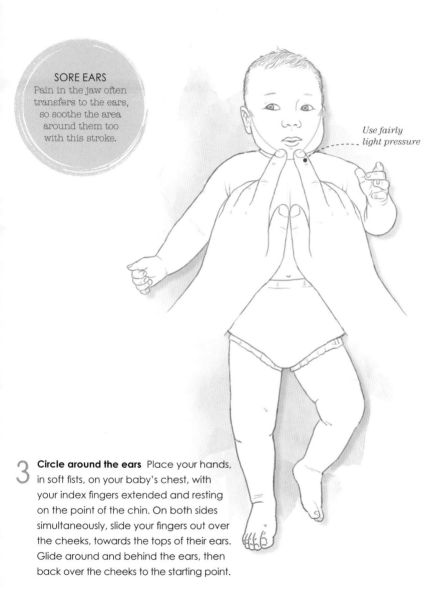

SORE EARS
Pain in the jaw often transfers to the ears, so soothe the area around them too with this stroke.

Use fairly light pressure

3 **Circle around the ears** Place your hands, in soft fists, on your baby's chest, with your index fingers extended and resting on the point of the chin. On both sides simultaneously, slide your fingers out over the cheeks, towards the tops of their ears. Glide around and behind the ears, then back over the cheeks to the starting point.

97

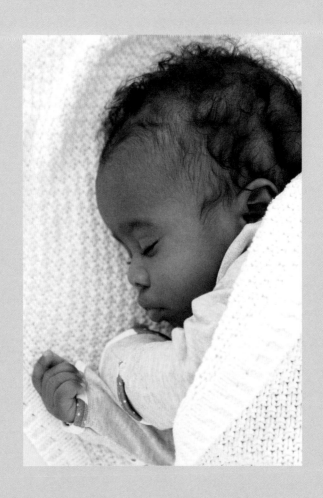

"Even just a few minutes of massage can be wonderfully relaxing for both giver and receiver."

CONGESTION

If your baby gets a cold, use these simple strokes to comfort them while holping to shift mucus in the lungs and drain the sinuses. Massage will also give your baby's immune system a boost to fight infection.

Babies can get up to ten colds a year before they reach the age of two. This is because their immune system is still developing, and they have yet to build up resistance to different viruses.

Massaging your little one when they have a cold can be helpful for a number of reasons. Massage strengthens the immune system, helping your baby fight off infections; it will also calm and comfort your baby, easing the distress caused by difficulties in breathing or sleeping.

CLEARING CONGESTION

If your baby has a blocked nose, gently stroking their face will encourage mucus in the sinuses to drain away (see step 3). Sometimes babies also become congested in their chest; if your baby is coughing, the first two strokes in this sequence may help to clear out excess phlegm from their lungs. If your baby has a temperature, don't do any massage – you'll risk upsetting them further. Always consult your GP if you have any concerns about your baby's health.

These strokes work best if your baby is unclothed, although the "raindrops" technique can be done over clothing and does not require oil. Do these strokes with your baby either lying down on their back or, if it's more comfortable for them, sitting up. If they are lying down you may wish to place something soft, such as a pillow or blanket, under their head to raise it slightly and make them more comfortable.

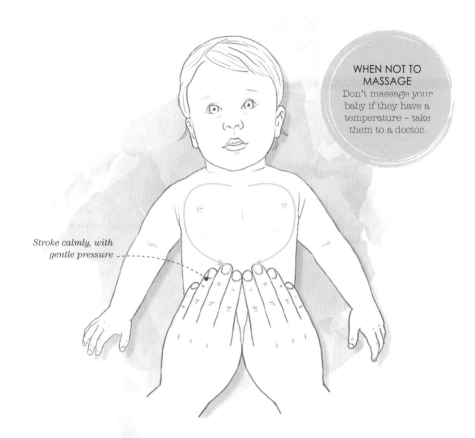

Stroke calmly, with gentle pressure

1 **Draw a heart** Place both hands over your baby's chest, fingers resting on their collarbone. Slowly slide your fingers out to the shoulders and down the torso, bringing them together at the base of the breastbone. Then glide back to the starting point. This warms up the area, relaxes the chest and ribcage, and loosens phlegm.

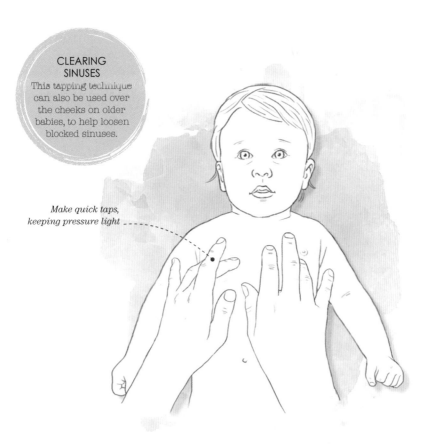

CLEARING SINUSES
This tapping technique can also be used over the cheeks on older babies, to help loosen blocked sinuses.

Make quick taps, keeping pressure light

2 **Make "raindrops" on the chest** Use your fingertips to tap lightly all over your baby's chest, especially over the ribcage, for a minute or so. This will help to loosen phlegm, so it can be coughed up more easily.

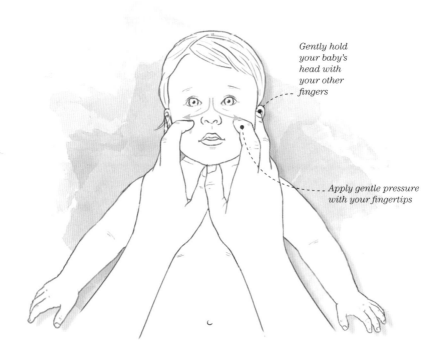

Gently hold your baby's head with your other fingers

Apply gentle pressure with your fingertips

3 **Stroke down the nose and out over the cheeks** Steady your baby's head by placing your hands on either side of their face. Bring your index fingers to the bridge of your baby's nose. Now slide your fingers down the nose and out over the top of the cheekbones. Repeat several times.

SKIN CONCERNS

It's perfectly normal for babies' skin to become dry, flaky, or reddened as they adapt to the outside world. While massage alone can't directly heal skin concerns, it does help to reduce stress and nourish skin from within.

We all want our babies to have beautiful, healthy skin, but sometimes they develop dry patches, eczema, or an intolerance to something that may show as a skin complaint. Our skin is the largest organ in our bodies, and the one through which we have the most direct interaction with our environment. It's quite normal for newborn babies' skin to go through a stage of spottiness or dryness, or even to have flaky patches, as they adjust to their surroundings.

SOOTHING WITH TOUCH

Many skin problems are brought on, or made worse, by stress – the same is true for babies. Since massage is an effective way to reduce levels of the stress hormone cortisol, it can also help treat skin conditions. Studies have shown that when a moisturiser is mindfully applied via massage it has a more beneficial effect than it would if it were simply rubbed into the skin.

When massaging your baby, use a cold-pressed vegetable oil. It is best to avoid artificial aromas – often listed as "parfum" in the ingredients list – and additives. Keep what you put on your baby's skin as natural as possible (see page 14). If your baby has dry skin, you may wish to use more oil than you normally would.

WHEN AND HOW TO USE MASSAGE

You can use the full top-to-toe routine (see page 18) to soothe your baby when they have skin issues, or just perform part of the routine if you prefer. Don't massage any areas of skin that are cracked or weeping. You may also wish to avoid any areas that are particularly inflamed or red if you don't feel comfortable massaging them.

If your baby shows signs of distress or discomfort during the massage, stop immediately, and do not continue. If you have any concerns about your baby's skin always consult your health visitor or GP. While massage can help to ease some common skin complaints, it is not a substitute for proper medical care.

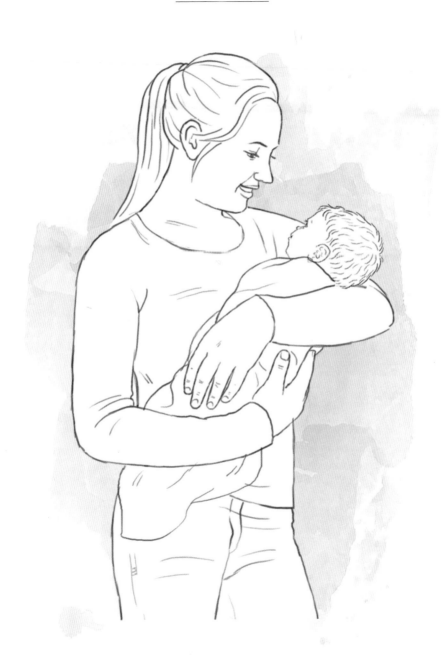

BEYOND
BABY

BEYOND BABY

This chapter allows you to explore massage further as your baby grows into a toddler and beyond. If you and your child still enjoy massage, there's no reason not to continue.

ADAPTING THE ROUTINE

Before you know it, your baby will be taking their first steps, learning to talk, and exploring the world around them. That doesn't mean they won't still benefit from massage, though. Massaging your child as they grow is mostly about adapting what you already know. You will find that as they get older it will become easier to communicate with them about which strokes they like best – but it might be trickier to get them to stay still long enough for a massage.

If you're massaging a wriggly toddler you may find you have to change the routine you are used to, but do continue if you can. As they get older, you will be able to return to the full top-to-toe routine, and in time they may even want to massage you!

MASSAGE FOR OLDER CHILDREN

The tummy sequence (page 30) in particular is a great one to continue as your baby grows. We all hold tension in our tummies when we feel anxious, and children will often say they have a tummy ache when in fact they just feel a little stressed or worried. A gentle tummy massage at bedtime can lead your child to open up and talk to you about their day, encouraging communication and re-establishing a loving connection.

If you have another baby, try involving your older child when you massage them, to share the importance of gentle, loving contact. Massaging your little one through their childhood teaches them the value of positive touch – and there is nothing better than when they want to massage you in return!

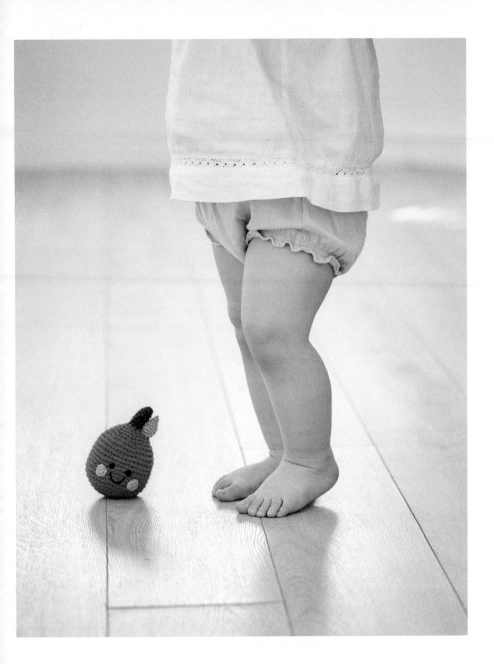

TODDLERS

Once babies are on the move, their muscles grow and change quickly. Massage will support your toddler's development, both physical and emotional – if you can get them to stay still long enough.

WHEN TO USE
Before bed, or whenever you like

GOOD FOR
Supporting muscle growth and encouraging relaxation

For a toddler who is more interested in exploring than lying still, getting through a full massage routine may prove difficult. If you've been massaging your child since they were a baby, though, it is worth persevering with your usual massage routine – they will invariably come back to it, and may even ask for a massage.

STARTING MASSAGE WITH A TODDLER

If you are new to massage, your toddler may respond well to the strokes on the next few pages; you can then build up to using all the strokes in the baby section, as your toddler gets used to it. If you find that your toddler doesn't take to massage, don't worry – try again when they are a bit older, and you may find they have changed their mind.

Right before bed is the ideal time for a short routine such as this. Bring your bedtime routine forward a little to incorporate a massage. You may only spend 5 or 6 minutes doing the massage, or it could last 20 minutes – your toddler will definitely tell you when they've had enough!

COMMUNICATION

Be guided by your toddler during the massage; ask if they want more or less, a stronger or lighter touch, and so on. This is the perfect time to practise rhymes or singing, which babies and toddlers love to hear. Use songs or rhymes they know and that have a body connection – *Heads, Shoulders, Knees and Toes* or *This Little Piggy*, for instance – to make it fun!

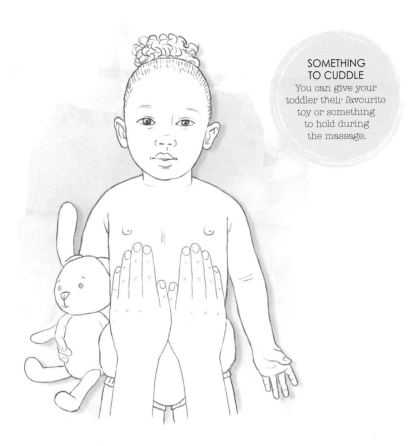

SOMETHING
TO CUDDLE
You can give your
toddler their favourite
toy or something
to hold during
the massage.

1 **Massage the front of the body** Ask
your toddler to lie on their back. Place
your hands over their chest, fingers
resting on their collarbone. Stroke
down their body, over their legs, and
right down to their toes. Repeat
several times, alternating with stroking
down the arms and over the fingers.

Continued... **111**

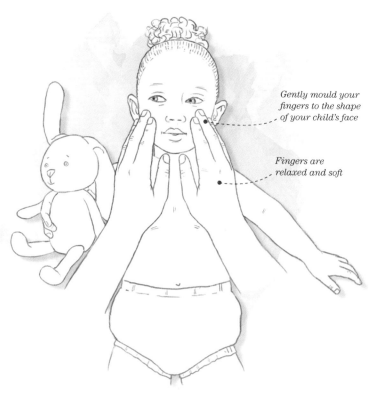

Gently mould your fingers to the shape of your child's face

Fingers are relaxed and soft

2 **Stroke the face** Cradling your toddler's head in your hands, softly stroke over their cheeks around the eyes and smooth their forehead. Lower your hands to make circular strokes over the middle of each cheek, simultaneously.

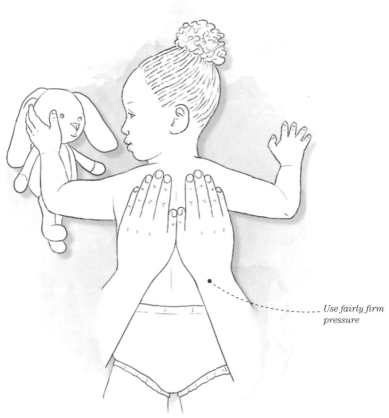

Use fairly firm pressure

3 **Massage the back of the body**
Ask your toddler to lie on their tummy. Place your hands over their shoulders on either side of their spine. Stroke down your toddler's body, continuing over the legs and right down to the feet.

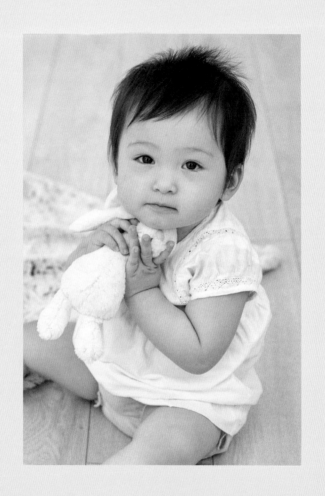

" We all need positive touch to thrive – and massage is the perfect way to connect with your child skin-to-skin. "

OLDER CHILDREN

As your child grows, you can continue to massage them with the routines you used when they were a baby or use these strokes for a quick massage to help your child feel calm and loved, and encourage communication.

WHEN TO USE
Bedtime, or whenever
you like

GOOD FOR
Encouraging
communication, teaching
your child about
positive touch

ADAPTING MASSAGE

The baby massage sequences given in this book will also work well for older children. Adjust the strokes as you go and focus on their favourite parts! You can adapt strokes and make them personal to suit your child's daily experiences, be it school or nursery, or a more physical activity like gymnastics or football. Explain how the massage helps to soothe and relax their muscles after a busy day.

Bedtime is always a good time to introduce some soothing touch. Massage can help to encourage a dialogue about how your child is feeling, as well as being an effective way to help your child relax before they go to sleep.

INCLUDING OLDER SIBLINGS

With the arrival of a new family member your firstborn will need time to adapt to their new sibling. They may watch you doing a massage on their new baby brother or sister and feel very left out! If you did massage with them when they were a baby, you can tell them that, and it may give you an opportunity to re-establish massage time with them.

You could also suggest that they massage a favourite doll or teddy (without using oil) while you massage the baby. Or, under supervision, the older child may want to massage their younger sibling as you guide and assist.

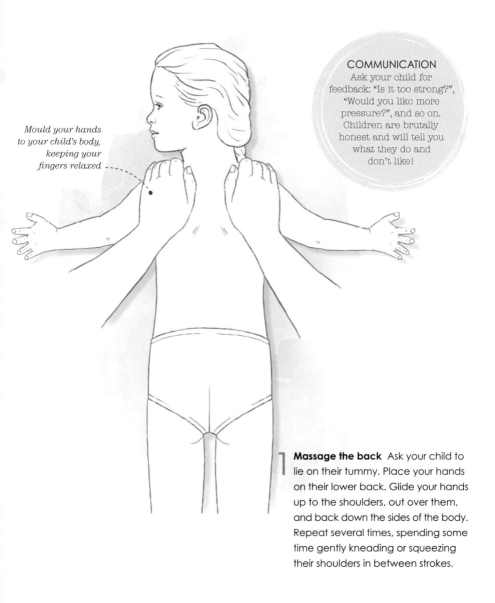

Mould your hands to your child's body, keeping your fingers relaxed

COMMUNICATION
Ask your child for feedback: "Is it too strong?", "Would you like more pressure?", and so on. Children are brutally honest and will tell you what they do and don't like!

1 **Massage the back** Ask your child to lie on their tummy. Place your hands on their lower back. Glide your hands up to the shoulders, out over them, and back down the sides of the body. Repeat several times, spending some time gently kneading or squeezing their shoulders in between strokes.

Continued...

**EASING
TENSION**
Children find tummy
massage soothing, as they
often hold tension in this area.
Massage here helps them
relax and may provoke an
outpouring of thoughts
and feelings.

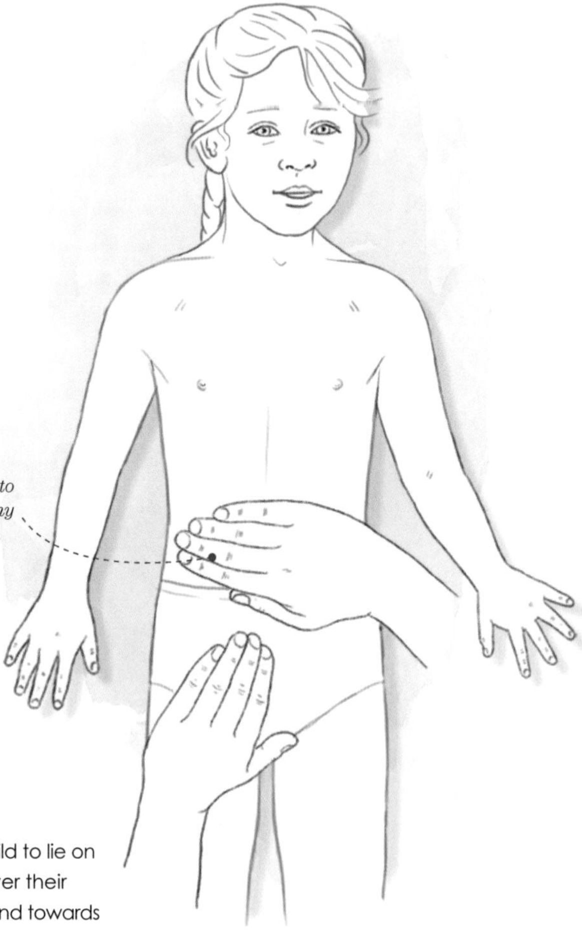

*Mould your hands to
the shape of the tummy*

2 **Stroke the tummy** Ask your child to lie on
their back. Place one hand over their
tummy and pause. Slide the hand towards
the groin, placing your other hand on
the tummy. Do this continuously a few
times, alternating hands. Then use one
hand to circle the belly button in a
clockwise direction. Repeat 5 or 6 times.

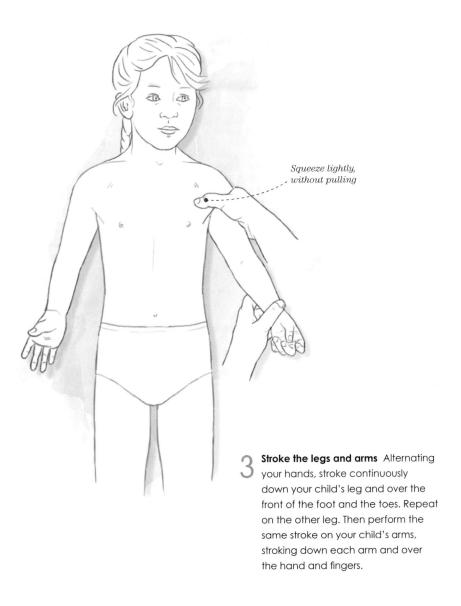

Squeeze lightly, without pulling

3 **Stroke the legs and arms** Alternating your hands, stroke continuously down your child's leg and over the front of the foot and the toes. Repeat on the other leg. Then perform the same stroke on your child's arms, stroking down each arm and over the hand and fingers.

SPECIAL
SITUATIONS

SPECIAL SITUATIONS

If you find you are faced with challenges beyond what you expected when your baby arrives, massage can be an especially therapeutic way to communicate love and reassurance.

MASSAGE IS FOR EVERYONE

Adapting to life as a parent – and establishing a bond with your baby – can be challenging, especially when the unexpected happens. If your baby arrives early, for instance, or has special needs, you may experience a range of emotions that can be difficult to manage. The process of adopting a baby can also be exhausting and uncertain.

Massage can help in all these situations. It is calming, reducing stress for both you and your baby, and can help support babies with developmental delays by building communication, improving growth and development, and teaching body awareness.

INTRODUCING MASSAGE

The routines in this chapter are shorter sequences, designed to introduce your baby to massage in a gradual way. Feel free to work through the longer routines in this book as well, choosing what you think is best for your baby. However, starting slowly and with fewer strokes – which means less stimulation – can be a good way to begin.

Don't worry if you don't feel very confident to begin with. A loving touch is always a good thing; just holding or stroking your baby softly will bring them comfort and security.

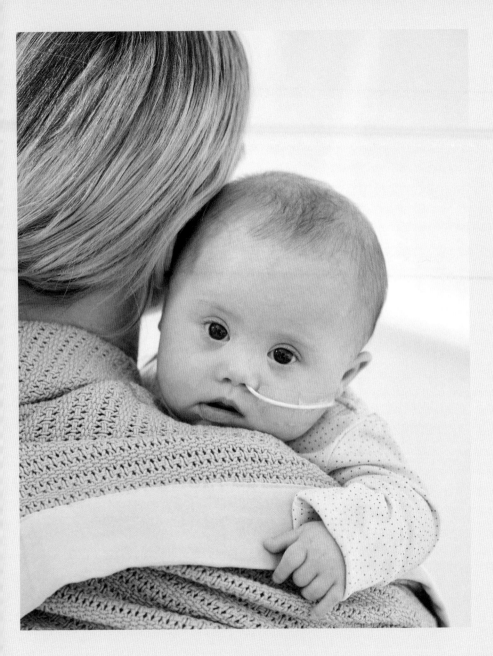

PREMATURE BABIES

If your baby is born prematurely, it may seem as though all your careful planning has been thrown up in the air. Massage can play a key role in helping the two of you to connect.

COMFORTING PREMATURE BABIES

If your baby arrives early, the bonding process may be delayed or different from what you expected. Because premature babies are still developing their body systems – changes that would have normally happened in the uterus – they are particularly sensitive. They will be exposed to medical procedures and equipment that may cause them distress and discomfort. The good news is that you can use modified massage strokes, guided by the medical staff, to comfort and bond with your baby even while they are still in hospital; some soothing touch will ease the wait to bring them home.

Your approach should be slow and extremely gentle. There may be areas of your baby that you will not be able to massage at first due to medical equipment, but even just hearing your voice and feeling your touch will bring comfort to your baby.

ADAPTING BABY MASSAGE

If you are ready to try massage, start with the area of your baby's body that has been the least traumatized, and at first only massage for a few minutes at a time. As much as possible, make sure you are relaxed; your baby will pick up on your emotions, so take a deep breath and know that what are you doing will bring them – and you – some relief.

Once home, you can continue down the path of exploring and developing a massage routine. If your baby is well enough, place them on your lap on top of a towel to massage them.

Because your baby is so tiny, you may need to use only two or three fingers to stroke your baby, rather than your whole hand. However, keep in mind that too light a touch can be uncomfortable and overstimulating for your baby, so keep all massage strokes fairly firm while still being gentle, as with the other sequences in this book.

Your baby will have experienced touch that has been invasive and very often painful – your main goal is to teach them that touch is a good thing. Talk to your baby in a soothing, loving way as you touch or stroke them, and stop the massage if they seem distressed.

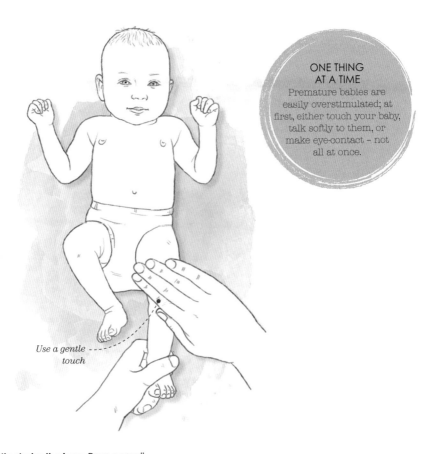

ONE THING
AT A TIME
Premature babies are
easily overstimulated; at
first, either touch your baby,
talk softly to them, or
make eye-contact – not
all at once.

*Use a gentle
touch*

1 **Gently stroke the legs** Pour a small
amount of oil into your hands and
warm it by rubbing them together.
Supporting your baby's ankle with one
hand, use your other hand to gently
stroke your baby's legs.

⟩ *Continued...* **125**

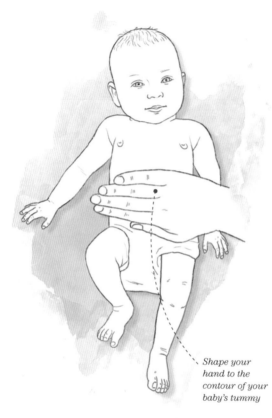

**ADDING TO
THE ROUTINE**
Once your baby is
stronger and used to being
touched, you can gradually
start to introduce other
massage strokes from the
top-to-toe sequence.

*Shape your
hand to the
contour of your
baby's tummy*

2 **Lay your hand over the tummy** Place
your hand lightly over your baby's tummy,
without too much pressure. Keep your
hand relaxed and rest it there for a minute
or two if your baby is happy.

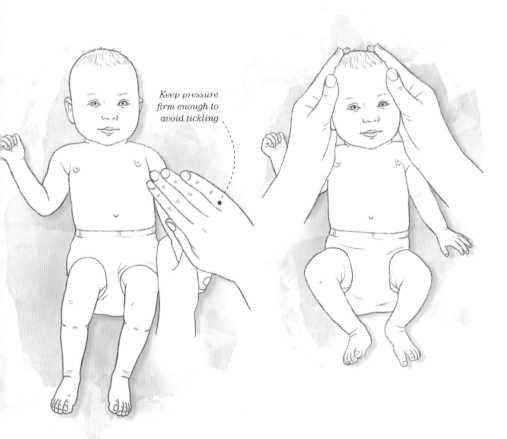

Keep pressure firm enough to avoid tickling

3 **Gently stroke the arms** Stroke along your baby's arms with one hand, supporting their wrist with the other. Observe your baby's reactions and stop or pause if necessary.

4 **Cradle the head** With both hands, gently cradle your baby's head. Even just holding parts of your baby's body will help them feel nurtured and loved.

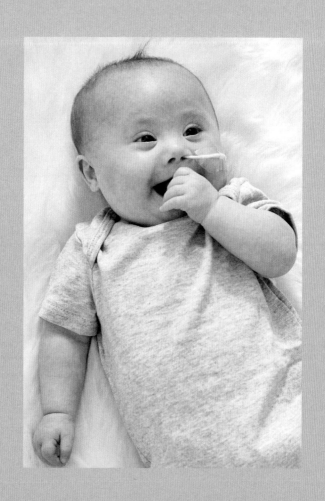

"Regular massages provide valuable moments of pleasure and relaxation for you both."

ADOPTED BABIES

If you're an adoptive parent, you may be particularly concerned about bonding with your new baby. Massage will show your baby they are loved and provide some much-needed relaxation for both of you.

PROMOTING LOVE AND RELIEVING STRESS

Making the decision to adopt a baby – and the subsequent process – can be long and fraught. You may feel overwhelmed and unsure, just like any other parent. Massage is a great way to connect with your baby and share some relaxing, loving moments together, reducing stress levels for both of you.

Be aware that some adopted babies may be developmentally delayed, and may not reach certain milestones as quickly as other babies. During what can be a stressful transition, some gentle, loving touch will work wonders at helping your baby feel calm, safe, and loved.

BONDING WITH YOUR BABY

Bonding is multi-faceted, but is mostly enhanced by touch, warmth, eye contact, smell, and vocal assurances. An adopted baby may not have experienced these things as much as usual during their early life.

Massage brings all these elements of bonding together, providing an opportunity for positive skin-to-skin contact that accelerates the bonding process, and allows you and your child to communicate non-verbally.

STARTING MASSAGE

When you feel ready to start massaging your baby, begin with just 5–6 minutes at a time. Tune in to your baby's signals and proceed with love. If your baby shows signs of distress, pause and let them know that they are safe and you are there for them. If there is a particular move that they don't like, leave it out until they are more used to the routine.

While you can of course work up to any of the routines in this book, it's best to start with a shortened routine to build the trust and love between you and your baby. The following sequence of strokes are a good way to get started.

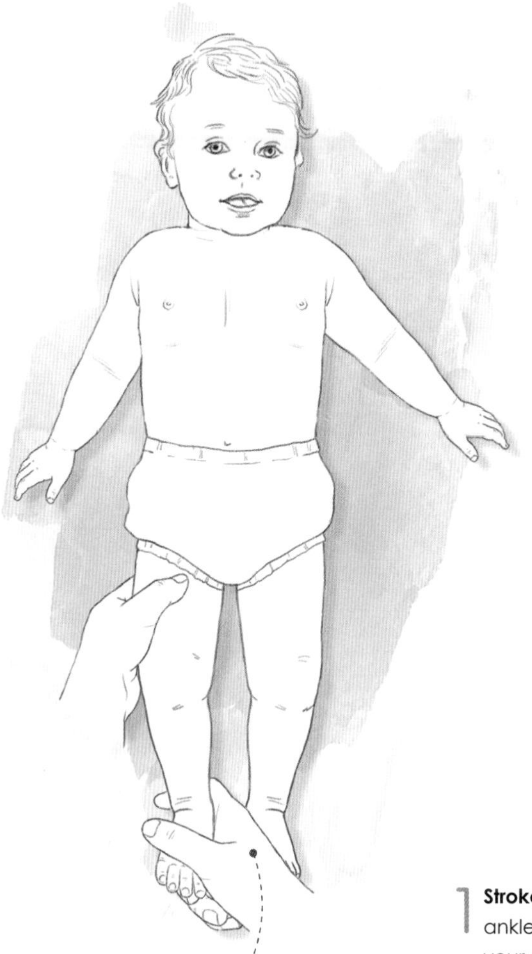

INTRODUCING
MASSAGE TIME
Try and build massage
into your baby's day in
a way that disrupts the
routine they're used to
as little as possible.

*Support your baby's
ankle with one hand
while you stroke
with the other*

1 **Stroke down the legs** Hold your baby's
ankle with one hand. Make a C shape with
your other hand and place it around the
upper thigh, thumb on top. Slide this hand
down the leg and over the foot, then stroke
your other hand down the other side of
the leg. Repeat several times, alternating
hands. Then do the same on the other leg.

❯ *Continued...* 131

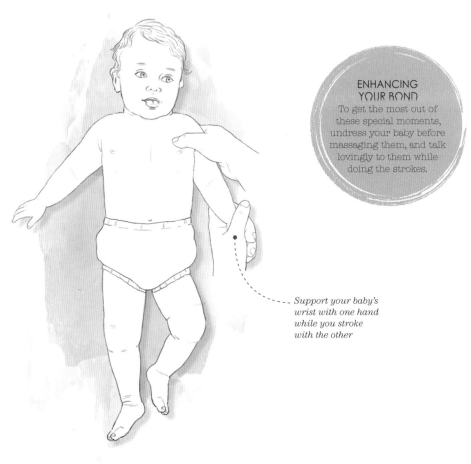

*Support your baby's
wrist with one hand
while you stroke
with the other*

2 **Stroke down the arms** Hold your baby's
wrist with one hand. Make a C shape with
your other hand and place it around the
upper arm, thumb on top. Slide this hand
down over the arm and hand, then stroke
your other hand down the other side of the
arm. Repeat several times, alternating
hands. Then do the same on the other arm.

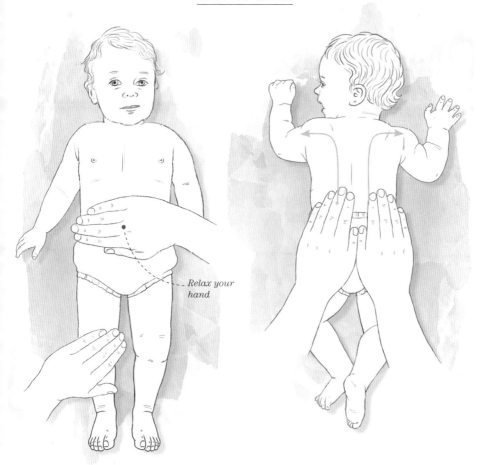

Relax your hand

3 **Stroke over the tummy** Place one hand horizontally over your baby's tummy and pause for a moment. Slide your hand down towards the groin, bringing your other hand to the starting point on the tummy. Stroke continuously over the tummy, alternating hands. Repeat 5 or 6 times.

4 **Do a T-stroke on the back** Place the palms of your hands over your baby's bottom, fingers pointing towards their head. Glide your hands up towards the shoulders following the line of the spine. Part your hands and stroke over the shoulders and down the side of the body, back to your starting position. Repeat several times.

BABIES WITH DISABILITIES

Touch is vital for everyone, and all babies will respond to positive contact.
Massage can be adapted to suit your baby's needs, then used to support
your child physically and emotionally as they grow.

COMMUNICATING LOVE

Coming to terms with and adjusting to a baby's needs is a huge part of parenthood. Adjusting to a baby with particular needs because of developmental issues or complications can be a more delicate transition. Massage will give you the opportunity to communicate with your baby, reassuring them and reinforcing your bond. If they have complicated needs, the soothing touch they receive during massage time will counteract any discomfort caused by medical procedures they may be experiencing.

READING YOUR BABY'S SIGNALS

Start slowly; it may be difficult to understand your baby's signals, so start with an area that is not too large, such as the legs. Gently stroke over your baby's body using slow, rhythmic strokes. If your baby has had surgery, work on areas of the body away from the operation site. If your baby has auditory or visual impairments they will likely respond to touch in a positive way, as their sense of touch will be heightened to compensate for the loss or impairment of other senses. Massage will help them learn about their body and feel more connected to you.

If your baby always shows a dislike for a particular move, miss it out! You are the best judge of your baby's needs. However, if they are under medical care, talk to their primary physician about incorporating massage into your daily life.

When you feel ready and your baby is enjoying the massage, you can add in any of the strokes from the full body routine that you think your baby will respond well to. To start with, though, the following strokes will provide a gentle introduction to the benefits of massage, for your baby and for you.

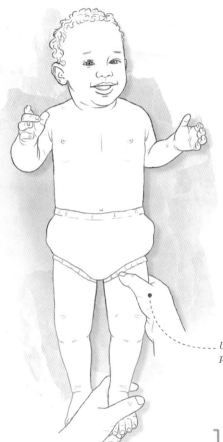

EXPERT
GUIDANCE
If your child has a
physiotherapist, speak
to them about the kind
of massage strokes or
movements that will
suit your child best.

*Use fairly firm
pressure but don't pull*

Stroke down the legs Support your baby's
ankle with one hand, and use your other
hand to stroke down their leg and over
their foot. Repeat several times, alternating
hands, then repeat on the other leg.

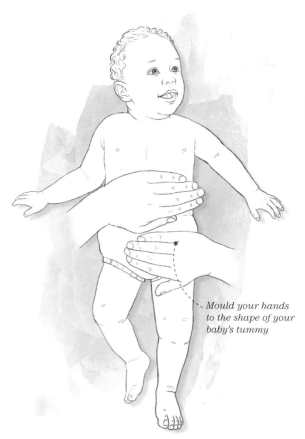

SKIN-TO-SKIN
CONTACT
This sequence will be
most beneficial if your
baby is naked.

*Mould your hands
to the shape of your
baby's tummy*

2 **Stroke over the tummy** Place one hand
over your baby's tummy and pause for a
moment. Slide your hand down towards
the groin, while bringing your other hand
to the starting point, then continue
stroking over the tummy, alternating
hands. Repeat 5 or 6 times.

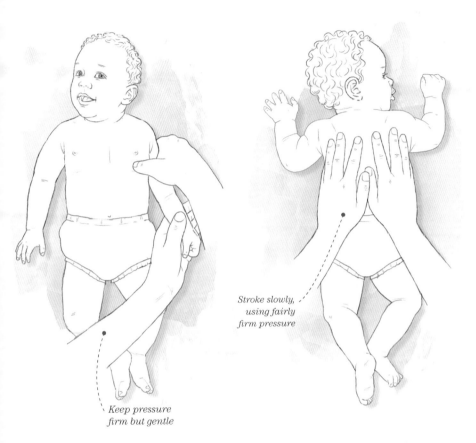

Stroke slowly, using fairly firm pressure

Keep pressure firm but gentle

3 **Stroke down the arms** Supporting your baby's wrist with one hand, use your other hand to stroke down their arm and over their hand. Repeat several times, alternating hands, then repeat on the other arm.

4 **Stroke over the back** Place your hands flat on your baby's back at either side of their spine, near the shoulders. Glide your hands down the back and over the bottom, continuing to the ankles. Repeat, then after a few strokes open your fingers to make this into more of a combing stroke. Repeat several times.

RESOURCES

There are a large number of organisations working to support and educate those caring for a baby. In addition to your health visitor and doctor, these resources may be of help.

BABY MASSAGE TRAINING

The International Association of Infant Massage
www.iaim.org.uk
An organisation that offers accredited training and qualifications in baby massage, as well as expert information for parents and massage instructors alike.

from the seed
www.fromtheseed.co.uk
Holistic aromatherapy and women's health practice run by Jo Kellett, which offers baby massage classes, both one-on-one and in groups, in Brighton.

NCT Baby Massage
www.nct.org.uk/get-involved/nct-training
Baby massage teacher training and the only university-accredited infant massage qualification are offered by the National Childbirth Trust.

GENERAL SUPPORT

National Childbirth Trust
www.nct.org.uk
A charity supporting parents through pregnancy, birth, and caring for a newborn. They offer courses and workshops (including those on baby massage), run local activity days, and provide extensive information on all stages of having a baby.

National Childbirth Trust Babies and Toddlers

www.nct.org.uk/baby-toddler
The branch of the NCT that offers advice specifically on caring for a baby or toddler.

Cry-sis

www.cry-sis.org.uk
Tel: 08451 228 669
A charity offering help and support to the parents and carers of crying or sleepless babies. Their hotline is open from 9am to 10pm seven days a week.

Mumsnet

www.mumsnet.com
An online forum for parents and carers to discuss all aspects of pregnancy, birth, and childcare.

SUPPORT FOR PARTICULAR SITUATIONS

The Multiple Births Foundation

www.multiplebirths.org.uk
An international charity working to support the parents and carers of twins, triplets, and more, and to provide specialist education and advice to healthcare professionals working with them.

INDEX

>Continued...

ABOUT THE AUTHOR

Jo Kellett is an aromatherapist and massage instructor based in Brighton, UK. Having received her Diploma of Holistic Aromatherapy from the Tisserand Institute in 1996, she ran a practice at the Portland Hospital in London, as well as a home practice, until returning to the Tisserand Institute to teach aromatherapy in pregnancy and essential oil therapeutics. Jo also trained as an infant massage teacher; this forms part of her holistic aromatherapy practice "from the seed", which focuses on women's health and pregnancy. Jo also teaches aromatherapy at Neal's Yard Remedies, London, and massage at The Institute of Traditional Herbal Medicine and Aromatherapy, as well as being Tisserand Aromatherapy's Essential Oil expert. She is a member of The International Federation of Professional Aromatherapists and a Certified Infant Massage Instructor.

ACKNOWLEDGMENTS

AUTHOR'S ACKNOWLEDGMENTS
Thank you to all the parents, carers and babies who have attended my baby massage course over the last 21 years – it's been a delight. Thanks also to the wonderful team at DK for their guidance with this book. Thanks to my partner, Richard, for his help and support. And thank you to the wonderful work and dediction of the IAIM, who encourage and teach the power of positive touch across the world.

PUBLISHER'S ACKNOWLEDGMENTS
DK would like to thank Rona Skene for editorial support, Louise Brigenshaw for key design work towards the end of the project, Kiron Gill for editorial assistance, Sarah MacLeod for proofreading, and Marie Lorimer for providing the index. Models: Aydin, Elizabeth, Maisie, Polly, and Ruby at Urban Angels.

DISCLAIMER
Before starting a massage on a baby, refer to the cautions on page 13. If you have any doubt as to whether or not to massage any part of your child's body, please consult your GP first. The information in this book has been compiled as general guidance on the specific subjects addressed. It is not a substitute and should not be relied on for medical or healthcare professional advice. Please consult your GP before changing, stopping, or starting any medical treatment for your child. So far as the author is aware the information given is correct and up to date as at 06/09/19. Practice, laws, and regulations all change and the reader should obtain up-to-date professional advice on any such issues. The author and publishers disclaim, as far as the law allows, any liability arising directly or indirectly from the use or misuse of the information contained in this book.

14/01/2020